Emotional

INFERTILITY

WORKBOOK

LEAH LLOYD

National Library of Australia Cataloguing-in-Publication data: Leah Lloyd/Emotional Infertility
Non-Fiction– Infertility

Editor: Natasha Gilmour
Proofreader: Teena Raffa-Mulligan
Cover and interior designer: Ida Jansson

ISBN: 978-0-6484803-7-2

NAME:

AFFIRMATION:

CONTENTS

Affirmations

I am not defined by my story.

Today I take back my power.

I have the ability to heal myself.

I connect with the healer within me.

I commit to showing my body unconditional love and gratitude every day.

I empower myself with knowledge.

There are many healthy changes I can make to help me have a baby.

It is safe to feel my emotions and to listen to what they are telling me.

I acknowledge and respect my feelings as I work through them.

I can choose to be the parent I want to be.

I take responsibility for my energy and my emotions.

It is safe to examine my emotions.

My happiness is my responsibility.

I remind myself to breathe…

I am worthy of a healthy and loving relationship.

Being a mother is my birthright.

I am grateful for all of the options available to me.

My past will no longer determine my future.

I can have a baby while respecting my culture and heritage.

I am deserving of more than one child.

I give myself permission to grieve my loss and to move on when I'm ready.

I am an equal partner in our fertility journey.

It is okay for me to feel a range of emotions now I'm pregnant.

With acceptance comes peace and I am okay.

Introduction

Emotional Infertility educates and empowers women (and men) through nineteen themed chapters with activities on how to assess where they are and how to cultivate their healing within. The *Emotional Infertility Companion Workbook* supports women (and men) on their journey with deeper considerations of each of those chapters through supplemental journaling, questions, tapping scripts, meditations and affirmations.

Make this companion workbook yours.

Write your name on the inside cover and underneath your name write your favourite affirmation from above. Say 'yes' to your path to heal infertility with all your heart.

With more than 100 pages of contemplative questions, affirmations, and plenty of space to write— by working through and addressing these issues, you give yourself the best chance of achieving a spontaneous pregnancy, or through assisted reproductive techniques, such as insemination or IVF. The goal of *Emotional Infertility* and this *Companion Workbook* is simply for you to look at some possible reasons why you may be experiencing infertility and identify any emotional causes behind them. We very rarely realise the effects our personal or learned beliefs have on our physical bodies, as well as the effects of the experiences that have led you to this moment. You may also find yourself coming back to sections of the book as different challenges arise for you on your journey. Each time you return to the book, you'll likely find that you receive different revelations depending on what's going on for you at that time.

I hope the process of reading *Emotional Infertility* and using this Companion Workbook will inspire your own realisations to heal and will serve you, whatever stage of the infertility journey you're on.

Before you begin,
I want you to know this: <u>It Is Not Your Fault</u>.

You didn't do anything wrong, and you don't 'deserve' infertility. If you are blaming yourself for anything, start to address it as you work through the activities—and learn and understand—helping you to make decisions that are right for you and letting go of what no longer serves you, beliefs, blame, guilt or anger.

If you are in a relationship and having fertility issues, it may be helpful to go through this process together. Sadly, relationships can break down during such a difficult time, and it is important to take steps to stay united in the process together.

My aim in writing this *Emotional Infertility Companion Workbook* is to give you the best opportunity to *emotionally* heal yourself. I'm sharing with you the processes that have helped my clients on their personal fertility journey. If you find you need more specific help with your emotions, please see a professional therapist. Emotions can become big and overwhelming particularly when going through something as significant and difficult as infertility, so it can be very helpful to have someone to talk through the process with.

There is no guarantee that by working through this process you will become pregnant. I wish I could give you that, but there are so many factors to fertility. This book will focus mostly on the *emotional* aspects. Seeing a fertility specialist and taking the appropriate steps with them may also be a vital part of this journey for you.

With over fourteen years of experience in nursing, I realised there was often more going on behind-the-scenes with conditions that weren't able to be identified or managed traditionally, leading to my interest in alternative therapies in infertility. To watch my weekly card reading videos, or to read the blog posts, go to:

www.facebook.com/LeahLloydHealer/ www.youtube.com/channel/UCbA5BLRdeUoVo9sjoZVibVQ

For further ongoing support, each month I send an email on a different topic and will include a variety of modalities, such as EFT, meditations, card readings, essential oils and other activities. For face-to-face or online forensic healing sessions you can see full details at www.leahlloyd.com.

Leah Lloyd

Before We Begin

"I commit to showing my body unconditional love and gratitude every day."

Before you begin, I encourage you to start your *Emotional Infertility* journey by watching the tapping script I have recorded for you, followed by a guided mediation *for body gratitude*—a powerful combination—to set your highest intentions towards your emotional healing.

Often when we are going through infertility, we start to blame our body for not working. This is a normal response, but it can be damaging if it lasts for a long period of time. We don't tend to look after something we don't appreciate. Our body is an amazing arrangement of intricate systems, that all need to work together to function effectively. Often it needs to do this with poor nutrient intake, high levels of stress, and unfavourable environmental influences. By using this meditation regularly, you will become more and more grateful for the body you have, and in turn will treat it better, which can only influence your *fertility* positively.

I guide you to read the *Emotional Infertility* book first, then come back to this *Companion Workbook* and take your time working through the pages. You may also need to re-visit some chapters as your journey unfolds.

Not everyone will read my books and go on to have a child, but I believe in my heart that many will. I hope these books can also bring you some comfort and healing.

Tapping The Healer Within

"I have the ability to heal myself."

EFT (Emotional Freedom Technique) fondly known as *tapping* is an incredibly easy technique to use. It is effective, free and you can do it anywhere. You can change the wording to suit your needs, or if you feel comfortable following the format I have created, make up your own script.

Before you start your first tapping session, spend a moment just sitting with your emotions—identify your stress levels from 0 to 10, zero being *no* stress and 10 being overwhelming stress. If you struggle to come up with a number ask yourself, 'do I feel less or more than an average stress?' then go above or below five. The actual number isn't so important, it's that the level of stress is decreasing as you tap that is important.

You will start with tapping 'The Karate Chop' point on the base of your hand down from your little finger. You will repeat the set-up statement or variations of the statement three times. From here you will move through the 8 points shown in the picture below saying your negative statements as you tap on each point. Do as many cycles of this as you need to until your stress is less than two, or the negative statements are no longer feeling true for you.

When you feel ready to move on, continue to tap through points 1-8 but start saying your positive statements. If they don't feel like you are being honest, you can add, 'I choose to…' or 'I wonder if…' or 'Maybe…' at the beginning. Keep going with the positives until you can lose these starting comments, or until they feel true for you.

Check in with how you're feeling when you think about the situation you just worked on. Is there any stress now when you think about it and if so, is it improved from before you started? Sometimes when you tap you start to think of other things that need to be addressed, other aspects of a situation or feelings you hadn't identified or acknowledged previously. This will likely be an ongoing process that you will need to revisit, but it's free, it's easy and it's really worth it, so stick with it.

Sometimes when we haven't been given a good education around something as important as our menstrual cycle, we can feel angry or hurt, creating emotional infertility blocks on our journey. Throughout this book, explore any issues that come up for you and use the tapping activity provided to process and create new beliefs, such as:

'I am empowered and have some control over what is happening.'

As you do the exercises throughout the book you will have a lot of information ready to use for your tapping. I find it useful to go through your answers and in one colour highlight the perceived 'negatives' and in another colour the 'positives'.

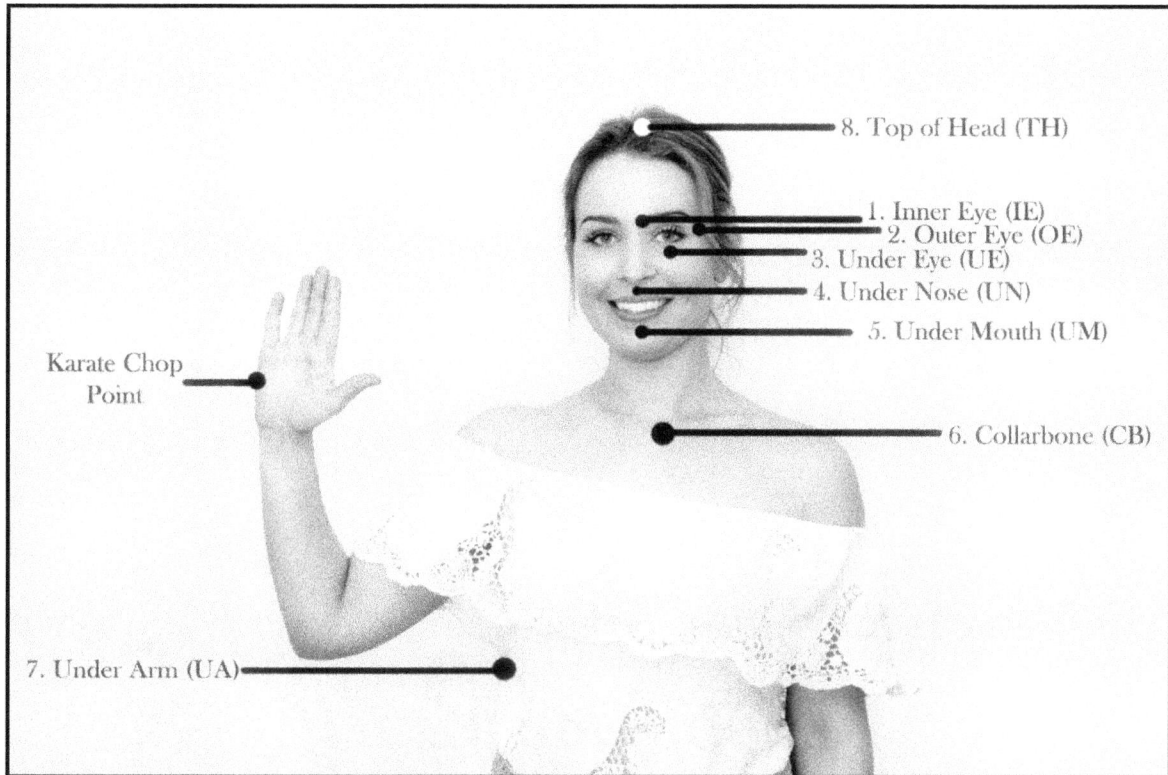

Where to tap

1. Inner Eyebrow (IE)
2. Outer Eye (OE)
3. Under Eye (UE)
4. Under Nose (UN)
5. Under Mouth (UM)
6. Collarbone (CB) *Use fist*
7. Under Arm (UA) *Use hand*
8. Top of the Head (TH)
9. The karate chop point (KP) *Use four fingers*

I Empower Myself
With Knowledge.

CHAPTER ONE
UNDERSTANDING YOUR CYCLE

Unfortunately, there is not an emphasis placed on education around women's bodies and how they work. There is an assumption that we are women, therefore we know. But in my experience, this simply isn't the case.

Here are the basics of a cycle:

The menstrual cycle begins with Day 1 of your bleeding, also known as a period, menstruation or menses, and continues until your next Day 1. This is normally 28-35 days in length and is usually quite regular. For some women however, it can be very irregular, ranging from days to months in length.

The menstrual cycle can be divided into four phases:

The Menstrual Phase – When a pregnancy does not occur in a cycle, the endometrium, or uterine lining, breaks down and results in a bleed. During menstruation, your oestrogen and progesterone levels are quite low and your ovaries are fairly inactive. If you are doing blood tests to track your cycle, you would likely be told 'everything is baseline' during this time. We consider the first day of your period, your Day 1 of the cycle. Your period usually lasts around 4-7 days, but this will vary between each woman, and different ages. The cervix is open during menstruation, and as the bleeding diminishes, the cervix closes and a mucous plug forms within it.

The Follicular Phase – Unless you are having a short cycle, you will experience a variable time of infertility after your period (yes, some people do ovulate during their period), while the follicles within your ovaries begin to develop. The cervix is closed with a mucous plug during this phase, which protects the reproductive system from infection and prevents sperm from entering. This stage will be dry with no mucous present, or some people experience a feeling of moistness with an unchanging type of mucous. Both of these are considered infertile. During the follicular phase, oestrogen levels rise, thickening the endometrium to prepare it for a pregnancy. Follicle Stimulating Hormone (FSH) also rises and assists to mature the eggs within the follicle. Generally, only one follicle will mature, but if more than one matures, this could result in a multiple pregnancy.

The Ovulation Phase – The developing follicles continue to produce oestrogen, activating the cervix to open and release the mucous plug, and produce the mucous essential for sperm survival. The presence of this mucous indicates fertility as this mucous nourishes and protects the sperm, maintaining their fertilising capacity for a few days, carrying the sperm through the cervix, the uterus and the fallopian tubes ready to connect with the ovulated egg. The pituitary gland triggers the release of a hormone called Luteinising Hormone (LH) which causes the mature follicle to burst, releasing the egg into a fallopian tube. When the egg leaves the follicle, the empty follicle becomes the corpus luteum, which produces oestrogen and progesterone and continues to thicken the endometrium and nourish an embryo if it is made. The mucous in this phase changes from a moist to a wet to a slippery sensation. The last slippery day signifies ovulation most of the time. Progesterone starts to rise just before ovulation, causing the thickening of the mucous, which creates the noticeable change in mucous sensation. Pregnancy is possible on all days when fertile mucous is present and for 3 more days past ovulation (this allows for the lifetime of the egg and late ovulation, which can be 2 days after the last slippery day). The egg has a lifetime of 12-24 hours after it is released from the follicle, in which time it needs to be fertilised to result in a pregnancy.

Sperm can stay alive for up to four days when fertile mucous is present, so sex in the lead-up to ovulation day can still result in a pregnancy.

The Luteal Phase – The Luteal phase begins the day after ovulation until the start of your next bleed. If the egg is not fertilised, it disintegrates, causing the oestrogen and progesterone levels to drop. The endometrial lining breaks away and a period occurs. This phase is typically 14 days but can vary from 11-16 days in a normal cycle. A short luteal phase does not allow for an embryo to implant and results in an infertile cycle. This is usually caused by a drop in the hormones prematurely following an ovulation problem. A long luteal phase suggests pregnancy or incorrect identification of ovulation.

So, how does this information help you to become pregnant?

For pregnancy to occur, the following things must happen.
- The ovary must release a healthy egg into the fallopian tubes.
- Healthy sperm needs to be in the vagina when the fertile mucous is present.
- The fallopian tubes must allow the egg and sperm to travel unobstructed.
- If fertilisation takes place, the embryo must arrive within the uterus when the endometrium and embryo are at the right stage for implantation.

In addition to this, you:
- Must be able to identify your fertile mucous.
- Must have intercourse when there is fertile mucous present.
- Have intercourse every second day during the slippery mucous if possible. A day off in between allows you to re-assess your mucous, so you can identify ovulation. Have intercourse at other times during the month too as you want to be replenishing the sperm, and this allows you to have intercourse with your partner at times when there is no expectation of pregnancy occurring. This is important for a relationship, so neither party begins to feel 'used' or like a 'baby making factory'.

1. Did you learn anything new about your cycle?

_____

_____

_____

_____

2. Is there information you knew or didn't know?

_____

_____

_____

3. Does this change things for you now as far as when you are having sex, or giving you more control over when you are likely to be fertile?

_____

_____

_____

_____

4. Do you remember when you had your first period?

_____

_____

_____

_____

How old were you?

_____

Did you know what it was?

_____

What were you feeling at the time?

_____

_____

_____

_____

Did you have support?

_____

_____

_____

_____

Are there any beliefs or experiences you are holding on to that you need to explore and process now?

_____

_____

_____

_____

_____

_____

_____

_____

5. What do you say about your period now? Is it painful and a nuisance or is it manageable? Explore the wording you use.

_____

_____

_____

_____

_____

_____

_____

_____

_____

_____

_____

_____

6. Start tracking your cycles. Write down the day your period starts, when it ends, when your slippery mucous starts and ends, when you believe ovulation to be, and how long between ovulation and your next period. This will give you so much information and will develop a connection with your body that you understand, and can support your body at the times it is needed. If you are trying for a baby right now, this could be the simplest thing you do to make that a reality.

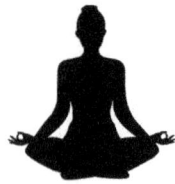

Meditation: for physical reproductive ailments

There is a lot of evidence to suggest the mind can have a great influence over the body and how it functions. This meditation focuses on clearing any reproductive system issues and bringing health and wellness to the reproductive system. There is a long relaxation in the beginning because this is vital to improving the effectiveness of the meditation and allowing the body to heal, so don't skip this part if it feels too long. Not all of the issues mentioned will apply to you, so if you're recording the meditation you might want to leave some parts out. This meditation is specific for women.

Just gently close your eyes. Take a few nice deep breaths. Just breathing in peace and starting to let go of any stress or tension that you feel within you. I want you to become aware of a vast space around you. A nice, dark, safe space. Surrounding your body. And as you open your eyes and look into this space, you notice in the distance, a rainbow light. Full of blues, and greens, pinks, purples, orange, red and yellow... and any other beautiful, vibrant colours that you need right now.

As the light comes closer, notice it appears to be dancing... swirling around... carefree and happy. The light starts to surround you... swirling around your body... the energy of the light lifts your arms and legs, until you feel like you too are dancing with the light. The light has a strong energy... an uplifting and empowering energy. And as you dance with the light, it enters your body through your feet, and swirls up your legs and trunk, lifting you with its energy, as it flows down your arms, and up into your mind. The rainbow light exits out your fingertips, and out of your crown chakra, and your feet, until your whole body is glowing with these beautiful rainbow colours. Enjoy the feeling that this brings. The strong, positive vibes that this rainbow light brings to your body. Feel your body move freely, there's no restrictions of time or space, as you dance as one with the beautiful rainbow light.

When you are ready, your body returns to stillness, the rainbow light settles in front of you, and it circles in a ball. You reach out with your hands cupped... outstretched in front of you, and the rainbow light ball sits comfortably within your hands, as though it belongs there... as if it is part of you. And as you watch the ball, gently rotate in your hands, you feel the strength and the energy in your hands.

Become aware now of your reproductive system that would benefit from the healing energy that you have now in your grasp. Feel in your body anywhere it is needed... it may be your ovaries, your fallopian tubes, your uterus... get a sense of which colour would best serve you at this time and see that colour coming out of the energy ball and into your fingers, though the palms of your hands and up your arms, and travelling to the part of your body where it is needed. See the colour starting in your ovaries... filling each ovary with healing light... gently healing any cysts... sending nourishing love filled light to your ovaries and the eggs within... when your ovaries feel healed allow the light to travel down each fallopian tube... clearing each tube as it moves through with flow and ease... gently dissolving any blockages you sense... as the healing light enters your uterus, allow it to spread throughout your womb... filling it with love... vitality... and health. See the lining thick, nourishing and welcoming to a future embryo... see the energy fill it with a vibrant, healthy colour...

Sit with the colour surrounding your whole reproductive system for a moment as it heals what is needed to be healed. As you relax and breathe, and let the colour do the job it has come here to do. It may be clearing blockages... calming overactive organs... or bringing life to those that need more vitality... you may need to bring in other colours or move it through to other parts of your reproductive system…

When the healing is complete, allow the colour to return back down your arms and out the palms of your hands or fingertips, back into the rainbow ball. And bring your attention to the rest your body and notice anywhere else that could benefit from the healing coloured light. Bring another colour from the ball through your fingertips or the palm of your hands and up your arms, and take it to where it is needed in your body. Allow that colour to swirl round where it is needed. To fill that part of your body, to fill it with its healing energy, and to provide that part of your body with anything else that it might need… so that your whole body is connected and functioning as one…

When it is complete, allow that colour to again return down your arms, and out your hands and allow it to again join that swirling energy ball in your hands.

You might like to imagine storing this ball of energy inside of you somewhere for safe keeping… Or perhaps there is somewhere around you that you know you can keep it, so it will be there when you need it again. Find that place now, for your ball of energy…

And when it is safe, and you feel ready, just bring your awareness back now to your breathing. Become aware of where your body meets the chair or floor. Feel the chair or floor hard beneath you, as you become aware of any sounds in the room… feel your body back in your physical body. You might like to wiggle your fingers and toes. And when you are ready… take some nice deep breaths… and when you feel you are completely back in your physical body you can open your eyes.

There are many healthy changes I can make to help me have a baby.

CHAPTER TWO
UNDERSTANDING INFERTILITY CAUSES

There are many factors in our lives that can impact fertility. Some of the most common causes are listed below with some healing guidance on how to begin aligning your emotional and physical ailments.

- **Stress and Anxiousness**

It could simply be the focus you are putting on trying to get pregnant—moving to a new house, a stressful day at work, illness or travel—any of life's stresses and daily duties can delay ovulation in your cycle.

- **Maintain a Healthy Weight**

It is recommended that women maintain a body mass index (BMI) between 19-29 to maximize chances of conceiving, and for men a BMI below 29 is important for sperm health. Obese women, particularly those with central obesity, are less likely to conceive per cycle. Obese women often suffer menstrual cycle disturbance and are up to three times more likely to suffer oligo-/anovulation. Weight management is best achieved through a healthy diet and regular exercise.

- **Diet**

A healthy and nutrition rich diet is important for pregnancy. In my experience, a Low GI diet or the Paleo diet have an incredible effect on the menstrual cycle, weight, general well-being and therefore fertility. You may want to consider reducing caffeine intake or eliminating sugar and grains from your diet. Do not starve yourself, this will affect your menstrual cycle, as well as your mental and physical well-being.

- **Exercise**

Overly-strenuous exercise has been found to be detrimental to fertility and hormone production, therefore a balanced and regular exercise program is recommended. Exercise is also good for your emotional well-being, which also improves your chances of conceiving.

- **Relationships**

It is vital to *not* put trying to have a baby before the health of your relationship. When intercourse becomes a chore or purely for the goal of conception, and is no longer about intimacy between partners, this will lead to strain on your relationship and increased stress.

- **Environmental Toxins**

Toxins are synthetic chemicals that surround us in our everyday life. They fill our cleaning products, skin and hair care products such as soaps, moisturisers, baby wipes, perfumes. They are in our food and water supply, in the soil, sprayed directly on the food, and in the water intentionally or as a bi-product. They are put in our furniture, carpet, plastic containers, cookware and clothing. The plastic toys our kids play with, the pages of the books they chew on, the receipts from the shops we go to and almost every single thing we touch. Over 80,000 chemicals are used in everyday products. Exposure to environmental toxins begins from the moment we are conceived. They cross the placenta and affect the development of the foetus. The issue is, our endocrine system either mistakes these chemicals for hormones, or they interfere with our hormones, and create havoc in our bodies. For example, BPA mimics oestrogen. So, in pregnancy the placenta filters natural oestrogen and prevents it from crossing into the foetus. However, while BPA has endocrine and oestrogen activity, it is not recognised by the detoxification enzymes, and they pass freely through the placenta to the foetus.

- **Smoking, alcohol or other drugs**

Smoking/passive smoking and alcohol are proven to severely harm pregnancy and lower sperm health. Some studies have found that women with a high alcohol intake take longer to become pregnant. Smoking is associated with an increased risk of miscarriage, bacterial vaginosis which is associated with late miscarriage, preterm labour, and with delivery of low-birthweight infants.

- **Age**

Statistically, fertility begins to reduce from the age of 35, reducing significantly after age 40. From the age of 45-49 the likelihood is less than 5% and falls progressively to zero after this. As you get older your cycles may become longer or more irregular, there are less fertile cycles, less mucous, and often shorter luteal phases.

Armed with this information, move on to the activities below.

Write down any reasons you are already aware of for your fertility issues. This may include lack of access to vital components, diagnosed medical conditions, physical issues, or any emotional reasons.

_____

_____

_____

_____

_____

_____

Do you have any of the issues outlined above?

_____

_____

_____

_____

Consider some other factors that perhaps could be affecting your fertility. What changes can you make now to positively impact your fertility?

_____

_____

_____

_____

_____

_____

_____

_____

_____

_____

_____

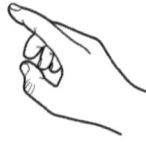

Tapping Script 1: for fear you did something wrong

When faced with infertility, a natural response is to question if you have done something wrong to create the situation. You might start to analyse your eating habits, your previous sexual partners, your sleep patterns, if that bath was too hot that time. It would be a good idea to explore these ideas before you start tapping so you can make your tapping script specific to you. Everything I have written here are examples of things I have been told by people or things I experienced myself. But I want to make it very clear to you, <u>this isn't your fault</u>, you haven't done anything wrong. I have deliberately left this script generic, so you can make it unique to you, so please put your own words in where "*xxx*" is written.

Karate Point (KP): Even though I'm starting to wonder if this infertility is my fault, I love and accept myself deeply and completely.

Karate Point: Even though I think I may have done something wrong to cause this, I love and accept myself deeply and completely.

Karate Point: Even if I did something wrong, I love and accept myself deeply and completely.

Inner Eyebrow (IE): I think this might be my fault

Outer Eye (OU): I think I caused it

Under Eye (UE): oh no, did I do this

Under Nose (UN): did my behaviour make this happen?

Under Mouth (UM): is it because I thought "xxx"?

Collarbone (CB) use fist: or because I did "xxx"?

Under Arm (UA) use hand: I always knew I would pay for that one day

Top of the Head (TH): that karma would come around

IE: I haven't always had the best diet

OE: I eat too much "xxx"

UE: sometimes I drink too much

UN: there were a few times I drank way too much

UM: did that cause this?

CB: there was that time I did "xxx"

UA: did that cause this?

TH: is this really my fault?

IE: I haven't always made the best choices

OE: with my health

UE: with my partners

UN: I haven't always been as nice as I could have been

UM: sometimes my emotions run away from me

CB: is this payback?

UA: is this karma?

TH: is this all my fault?

Keep going as long as you need to, being as specific to your circumstances and feelings as you can be.

IE: logically I know this isn't my fault

OE: but the fear remains

UE: I want to let it go

UN: I know this belief isn't helping me

UM: the fear keeps me stuck

CB: the guilt keeps me trapped

UA: it's time to let it go

TH: once and for all

IE: so, I am choosing to forgive myself

OE: for anything I did wrong

UE: for anything that may have contributed to this infertility

UN: I am choosing to love myself

UM: just as I am

CB: I am choosing to forgive myself

UA: for anything I may have done wrong

TH: and I am choosing to let this fear and guilt go

IE: it doesn't serve me any purpose

OE: other than keeping me stuck

UE: and I am choosing to not remain here

UN: I am freeing myself

UM: I am letting myself off the hook

CB: so, I can move forward

UA: I forgive myself

TH: <u>this isn't my fault.</u>

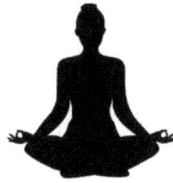

Meditation: for improving health

This meditation also has a long relaxation stage. Relaxing the body is vital for good health, and the deeper you can go into meditation the more effective it will be in creating long-lasting changes for you. Relaxation is key to a deep level of meditation. This meditation focuses on letting go of unhealthy patterns and behaviours and encouraging healthier lifestyle changes. This meditation is suitable for both men and women.

Find a comfortable position. You might like to sit in a chair with your feet firmly planted on the floor. Or you might like to lie down with a pillow and a blanket. Gently close your eyes and set the intention to take this time for healing…

Once you are comfortable, bring your attention to your breathing. Notice the breath coming in, and gently letting it out. You might like to deepen your breathing slightly, taking a deep, long, slow breath in to the bottom of your tummy, and gently let it turn and release it.

Begin to notice any stress or tension starting to leave with the out breath. Continue to breathe this way for a few moments. Just noticing your body starting to feel heavy against the floor or the chair… as you become aware of where your body meets the floor or the chair. Along your back, your bottom, your feet, allow them to sink in… notice any thoughts that come to you as you relax, and let them go…

Now notice the sensation of safe, comforting hands placed gently on your head. And where those hands meet your head, just feel the sensation of relaxing spread across your scalp, and down around your face. Feel your eyes gently closed and relaxed, not needing to see anything external at this time. Allow the relaxation to extend to your nose, along your cheek bones, as your face gently relaxes. Allow your mouth to relax now, there's nothing it needs to say or do right now. This is time just for you, just to be, just to relax…

Allow the sensation of relaxation to spread down over your ears, down over your neck. Just allow your neck to relax now and soften. Feel those comforting hands rest gently on both shoulders. Feeling the sensation of the relaxation extending across your shoulders, massaging in between your shoulder blades, allowing any tension… any knots… to start releasing. Feel the relaxation spread gently down your spine, relaxing… lengthening every vertebra, and allow the sensation to spread out to your ribs, become aware of the extension between your ribs as you breathe in… and as you gently breathe out let it relax, feeling any stress starting to go.

Allow the relaxation to spread around to the front of your chest, down both arms like a gentle massage… going over those muscles in the tops of your arms, down into your elbows, your lower arms… relaxing your wrists and all the bones in your hands, feeling each finger lengthening and relaxing.

Allow the sensation of relaxation to run down both your sides and across your tummy. Allow yourself to sink heavily… as you relax deeper and deeper into the meditation.

You might like to feel the hands go gently down your back and rest at your lower back, removing any stress or tension that you are holding there, and feel the relaxation spread from your lower back into your hips… your pelvis… into the tops of your legs that are busy holding us up all day long… now is the time to let them relax. Feel this calmness stretch further down into your legs, through your knees and down into your lower legs. Relax your ankles, both of your feet… imagine the relaxing hands holding both of your feet… as you feel where they connect to the floor. Feel them extend from here down through the floor, into the earth. Keeping your body safe and grounded for this meditation.

Now in your mind's eye see yourself standing in your home... notice how you look... if you're healthy... notice your weight without judgement, but simply awareness... as if watching yourself in a movie, see yourself move throughout your day... notice what you eat... if you exercise... any unhealthy habits you may have that you no longer want. See yourself go to work, or any other daily practices you attend to... are those things helpful to your fertility journey? Notice if they make you happy... healthy... As you watch yourself now, without judgement, notice one thing you would like to change to create a happier and healthier you... it might be eating better... it might be exercising... it might be letting go of unhealthy habits... now see yourself start to do this as your movie plays out in front of you... see yourself making that healthy change... see how your body becomes more vibrant and healthy as you make this change... see a glow around your reproductive system as it becomes healthier... better functioning... grateful for the changes you are making... see the people in your life supporting you... noticing the healthy changes and the difference in you... see yourself looking vibrant... healthy... happy... forgive yourself for any past habits or behaviours you had that weren't healthy... and send encouragement and love to yourself now for making healthy and long-lasting changes... spend a few moments now enjoying this feeling...

Bring this feeling back with you now, knowing this feeling is always within you... as you start to notice your breath once more... notice where your body meets the floor or the chair. Feel your body... your back, or your bottom or your feet touch the floor or the chair. And bring your awareness back into these body parts. As you breathe in feel your physical body start to awaken. Notice where your feet meet the floor and start to give them a little wiggle... bringing full sensation back into your feet and the rest of your body. Take some nice deep breaths in and let them out... allow yourself to feel present in your physical body and in the room around you. Continue to wiggle your toes... your fingers... and allow movement into the rest of your body. When you are ready you can open your eyes. You might like to stay sitting there for a moment, just recalling any guidance or insight that you received. And when you are ready, you can feel refreshed and rejuvenated, ready for the day...

*It is safe to feel
my emotions and
to listen to what they
are telling me.*

CHAPTER THREE
TUNING IN TO YOUR EMOTIONS

What if I was to challenge your story?

Sometimes our beliefs are so ingrained we don't ever question them, but if we can learn to, we can make great changes in our life. Consider these questions.

1. How many children did your mum, grandma, aunty and sister have? What stories have they told about it? Was it easy or difficult? Have you repeated these stories throughout your life? How does this relate to your current situation?

_____

_____

_____

_____

2. Do your friends have children? Have they had fertility issues? What have they told you about it? Does this affect you in any way?

_____

_____

_____

_____

3. What are *your* beliefs on your current situation with regards to finances, career, living situation, relationship etc?

_____

_____

_____

_____

_____

_____

_____

_____

_____

_____

_____

4. What are the beliefs of *those around you* on your current situation with regards to finances, career, living situation, relationship etc?

_____

_____

_____

_____

5. Write a list of all the beliefs you can think of that you have around fertility. Now go through this list and mark off the ones you feel are your beliefs, or if not, who they belong to. Can you consider there might be a different way of looking at it?

_____

_____

_____

_____

_____

_____

_____

_____

_____

_____

_____

_____

_____

_____

_____

_____

_____

_____

_____

_____

_____

_____

_____

_____

Next to each point on the list, write a new affirmation that accepts your current situation. Here are some affirmations for you to use or make up your own.

Belief:
"All the women in my family have trouble getting pregnant,
it's in our genes."

Affirmation:
*"I choose to create a new story for me,
where I am fertile and
become pregnant easily."*

Belief:
"I am in a same-sex relationship, and my friend casually told me
I had chosen not to have children because of this, maybe she is right."

Affirmation:
*"Regardless of who I love,
it is my birthright as a woman to be a mother,
and my child will be loved and cared for."*

Belief:
"I am single, so if I have a baby on my own, people will think I had a one-night stand."

Affirmation:
*"I am a strong and independent woman,
who is more than capable of being a single-mum,
and no-one but me needs to know my story."*

7. If any of your new affirmations don't feel 'true' to you, then you will need to do some more work on these to clear the beliefs. It would be helpful to write your affirmations down and place them somewhere you will see them every day, on the bathroom mirror is a great place for this. Repeat them to yourself morning and night.

_____

_____

_____

_____

_____

_____

_____

_____

_____

_____

_____

_____

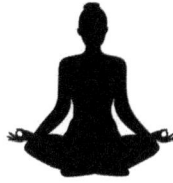

Meditation: for motherhood

This is a general meditation for seeing beyond infertility, to being pregnant and or being a mum. Often when the focus is only on getting pregnant, we don't consider how life will be after this point, and it can come as a big shock when we are pregnant or when we are a mum. This meditation is most suitable for women.

Find a place to sit where you are comfortable, and your back is supported. You might like a blanket to keep you warm. Take a deep breath in, down to your toes and gently let it go. As you breathe in, fill your body with peace, and as you breathe out, start to release any tension you are holding in your body... Becoming aware of your body as it presses against the chair or the floor. Notice your whole body, relaxing any areas of tension with every breath in...

Visualise a healing white light, entering your body from the tip of your head. Feel it light up your mind, your eyes, your ears, your nose, your mouth. Feel the light glide down the back of your head and around to your jaw. Let your jaw relax, and rest comfortably. Feel the light carry this relaxation down to your neck and across your shoulders and chest and upper back. The light flows down both arms, past your elbows, and into your hands and to the tips of your fingers. As the light fills your trunk, let it light up your heart, your lungs, your tummy, and your lower back. Feel the tension lift as the light travels down to your pelvis, through your hips, your knees, your calves and into your ankles and feet and toes. Feel your whole body relax now it is filled with this healing white light.

In your mind's eye, see yourself sitting comfortably as you look towards your stomach... you notice a baby bump... notice how this makes you feel... allow any emotions to come and sit with this as long as you need to... knowing your baby is safe within your belly... you might like to place our hands across your tummy as you connect with the baby within...

When you are ready move forward in time and see a much bigger tummy... you can feel your baby kicking now... again notice any feelings or emotions that come up for you... notice the people around you... those who are there to support you in this journey... see their smiling faces... see how loved you and your unborn baby are...

Again when you are ready move forward to the delivery of your baby... notice who is there to support you... a loved one, family or friends... the helpful doctor or midwife... everyone is supporting you and your baby as it arrives safely into the world... see yourself holding your baby for the first time... look in to your baby's eyes... you might be aware if your baby is a boy or a girl... you may even have a name chosen already... enjoy this time holding your beautiful healthy baby for as long as you like...

Moving forward in time when you are ready, see yourself at home, looking after your baby... notice how you look and feel without any judgement, send love to yourself for the great job you are doing... notice who is around to support you... see the beautiful connection you share with your child as you watch your baby grow into a toddler...

Spend as much time as you need to in this moment... notice any feelings or fears that may come to you... fill them with love and let them go... know you are safe, you are strong, you are a very good Mum.

When you are ready, start to notice the sounds around you, in the room where you are sitting, as you begin to settle comfortably back into your physical body. Become aware of your body and where your body meets the chair or floor. Become aware of your breathing, as you gently wake. Take some nice deep breaths in, and when you are ready, you can gently open your eyes, and sit still for a few moments, soaking in the feelings you experienced in this meditation.

You may like to journal these thoughts and feelings, or any insights that came to you. If you experienced any fears or uncomfortable feelings, journal these to work through later.

*I acknowledge and
respect my feelings
as I work through them.*

CHAPTER FOUR
HOW FEELINGS AFFECT FERTILITY

Usually when you start thinking about having a baby, you begin to notice babies everywhere. You smile at them and feel that stirring in the pit of your stomach, where you plan to have a baby of your own someday soon. All of your friends start having babies and you love to visit and buy them things, imagining that time in the not too distant future when you will be shopping for your own baby.

Nonetheless, time goes on ... and you don't become pregnant. And all of a sudden, those babies you see everywhere, and your happy mum-friends become a painful reminder of what you do *not* have, and what you may never have.

Before you move on to this activity, I want you to experience a happy emotion, so you can recognise the difference in your body. Imagine holding the baby you love in your arms, knowing everything is perfect. Your baby is healthy, you are healthy, your partner if you have one is happy, everything is good, you are safe to feel happy. Where is happiness in your body? You probably have a smile on your face. You might have tears in your eyes, but this will feel different to the tears of sadness. You will likely feel a warmth in your chest, your heart beating slow, steady and strong. Your arms and legs will most probably feel relaxed and free. You might feel a lightness you haven't felt for a while, like you can breathe again, the weight of the world that was on your shoulders now gone. This is the feeling you want to aim for when doing your healing work. Recreating how you will feel holding your newborn baby is the goal of using affirmations and doing your tapping.

1. Allow yourself an hour for this activity where you will not be interrupted. Sit where you are comfortable. Ask yourself the following questions and answer them as honestly as you can. Write as much as you need to so that you feel you have 'got it all out'. Write in the way you feel, use childish language, swear words, be resentful, bitter, angry, hurt—whatever you are feeling is what you are feeling—and that is okay. This activity is for you, and no one else.

Writing prompts:

Think back to the first time you imagined being a mum.

How did you feel?

What did you imagine it would be like?

How many children did you plan to have?

Were they boys or girls?

Did you name them?

Did you imagine being in a relationship?

What was that like?

How did you imagine your pregnancy to be?

What was the labour like in your imagination?

Had you thought of these things?

What was the future of your children like?

Did you see them growing up? Going through school? Graduation? Careers? Husbands/wives/children of their own?

Write it all down, every last detail.

Enjoy this feeling for a while, knowing it is still within reach.

_____

_____

_____

_____

_____

_____

_____

_____

_____

_____

_____

_____

_____

_____

_____

Now, think about the first time you thought you could be pregnant and found out you were not. This may not have happened yet, happened only once or many, many times. Write about these and how it made you feel.

Writing prompts:

How you feel about seeing other people with children, what your thoughts and opinions are of them?

How have these changed from your original opinions?

How you react to baby clothes or baby products in shops.

Who do you blame for not being pregnant? Yourself, your partner, God, your body, someone or something else?

Write all of this down, in as much detail as you can.

_____

_____

_____

_____

_____

_____

_____

_____

Sit with these emotions for a while, know it is okay to feel all of this.
Cry if you need to, scream, shout, hit a pillow. Just get it out of your body!

Now go through everything you have written and highlight the important parts. The words or feelings you can see that are not conducive to getting pregnant and welcoming a baby into your body or life.

In this table, write in the left column all of the words or statements you have highlighted. Now, next to these, write new beliefs. Note if these don't feel 'true' to you, you can start them with "I choose to feel…" as this may be easier for your body to believe, plus it gives you some power back over your feelings. Read over these new statements every morning and night. Cross them out once you no longer feel you need them. Add to them when something new arises. Change the wording as your experience and beliefs change. Remove the 'I choose to…' when you start to really believe the statements.

EXAMPLE:	NEW BELIEFS
I feel like my heart is breaking every time I see baby food at the supermarket	**I choose to look at the baby food and imagine which ones my future children will enjoy.**
I hate this useless body for not being able to get pregnant.	**I keep my body strong and healthy with good food and exercise and thank it for the baby it will one day carry.**
My friends get pregnant at the drop of a hat and they don't even appreciate it!	**I don't know anyone else's story, but I am happy for my friends when they have babies, and trust that my turn is coming soon.**

	NEW BELIEFS

	42

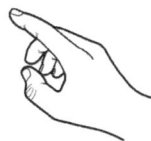

Tapping Script 2: for jealousy of other people having babies

This is a really difficult one, especially when it's your closest friends or family that are having the babies. It is easy to fall into the trap of feeling resentment, anger and jealousy. Often this leads to you also feeling a whole lot of guilt for having those feelings. You end up with a cocktail of emotions swirling around, changing from one second to the next and leaving you completely overwhelmed and upset. Remember it's okay to feel these things, but you want to put the time and effort in to processing them and working through them instead of taking it out on the people you love around you. It's not always easy but try to remember how you would want them to react if you announced you were the one having a baby and they were still infertile.

Karate chop (KP): Even though I feel jealous of those around me, I love and accept myself deeply and completely.

Karate chop: Even though I'm struggling to feel happy for others, I love and accept myself deeply and completely.

Karate chop: Even though I'm so angry right now, I love and accept myself deeply and completely.

Inner eyebrow (IE): It's so unfair

Outer Eye (OE): why do they get to have babies when I don't?

Under Eye (UE): are they more deserving than me?

Under Nose (UN): look at them flaunting their big tummies

Under mouth (UM): it makes me so angry

Collarbone (CB) use fist: I am so angry

Under Arm (UA) use hand: all of this anger in my body

Top of the head (TH): I feel like I might explode

IE: going to these baby showers

OE: it's killing me

UE: pretending to be happy

UN: when I just want to scream

UM: why them?

CB: why not me?

UA: what did I do wrong?

TH: I can't take much more

IE: I know it's not their fault

OE: but this hurts so much

UE: that's why I hold on to my anger so tightly

UN: because otherwise I will just feel sad

UM: and that sadness might kill me

CB: I can't take the sadness

UA: it feels like giving up

TH: at least with anger there's still a chance

IE: I'm still fighting for it

OE: I don't want to give up

UE: but it's so painful to keep wanting

UN: and to keep going without

UM: and I'm constantly being reminded

CB: by everyone around me

UA: baby showers

TH: talking about their kids in the lunch room

IE: I don't want to know

OE: can't they see they're hurting me?

UE: every time they mention their pregnancies

UN: or their children

UM: I hate it

CB: I hate feeling this way

UA: I feel so much guilt for feeling jealous

TH: I don't want to feel like this anymore

Keep going as long as you need to, being as specific to your circumstances and feelings as you can be.

IE: I need to start taking care of me

OE: all of this anger and hurt isn't helping me

UE: it doesn't help my body to have a baby

UN: I don't want to be this person anymore

UM: I want to be supportive of my friends

CB: but I can choose to not be around it all the time

UA: I can say no when I'm not feeling strong enough

TH: I give myself permission to take care of me first

IE: my friends will understand

OE: and if they don't that's still okay

UE: because my health is important

UN: and I am the only one that can look after it

UM: so, I am choosing to put me first

CB: and when I'm feeling good

UA: and strong

TH: I can be around my friends and their babies

IE: I have tools I can use

OE: I can tap before I see them

UE: I can journal how I'm feeling

UN: I can process the guilt rather than let it consume me

UM: I can feel the anger then let it go

CB: I can feel the hurt because I'm hurting

UA: I give myself permission to feel all of these things

TH: but I trust that I will be okay.

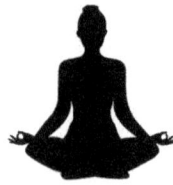

Meditation: for feeling joy when you see a baby

When we have been trying for a baby for some time and not getting pregnant, it can become very difficult to see other people with their babies, or to pass through the baby section of a store. This meditation focuses on recognising those emotions and helping to clear them, so you can find joy in spending time with other people and their children. This meditation is suitable for men and women.

Find yourself in a comfortable position. Allow your body to relax into the chair. Soften your shoulders... Have your feet sitting firmly on the ground, keeping you strong but comfortable. Become aware of any sounds around you within the room... Any smells you might notice... allowing them to bring you comfort in this journey. Take your awareness further outside of your room now... and become aware of any sounds outside... Perhaps there's traffic or birds... let the sounds just drift off into the distance, as you bring your attention to your body.

Now feel a white light travel down over your head... bringing with it peace and love and relaxation. Feel it going across your eyes as you let them relax... comfortable and peaceful. Down over your nose and across your cheek bones. Feel the white light relax your jaw and your mouth... It doesn't need to do any work at the moment, and it can take this time just to relax and re-energise. Feel the white light travel down over the top of your head and the back of your head... into your neck. Relaxing your ears... they only need to concentrate on my voice for this time, everything else can wait.

Allow your throat to soften... there's nothing you need to be able to say right now. Feel the white light go into your back, between your shoulder blades... massaging out any tension that might be held there. Feel the white light travel across your chest... into your shoulders, relaxing the joints. Down through the muscles of your arms, past your elbows... and down into your wrists and your hands. Let your arms feel heavy, as your hands gently rest in your lap or down by your sides. Allow the white light to relax the trunk of your body as it gently drifts around you, down through your back... relaxing your spine. Feeling it straighten and then soften gently against the chair or floor.

Let your tummy relax... and if you are holding any knots or tension there, allow it to start to dissolve as your body becomes heavier. Breathe down into your body, deep into your tummy... bringing oxygen into your tummy through the white light, so that it can relax.

Bring the white light down through your legs, through your knees... as they feel heavy against the chair or floor. Take a deep breath, bringing oxygen all the way down to your feet, and into your toes. Just notice if there are any other areas of tension in your body that need to be relaxed for this meditation, and bring the white light to those areas. Breathe in oxygen to those body parts that need it now... allowing your body to feel heavy, relaxed and peaceful.

Now in your mind's eye see yourself sitting in a quiet shopping centre... it's early and no-one else is there yet as you wait for the shop to open... as you sit there notice any thoughts that come, acknowledge them and let them go... as you sit there a lady begins to walk towards you with a baby in a pram... notice how this sight makes you feel... there's no judgement here, just simply allow the feelings to come... there's no right way to feel... just feel... allow your emotions to flow freely... let them out... send love to yourself at this time... and if it feels okay to do so, send love to the lady and her baby... knowing your time will soon come and the love you send out in to the world will flow back to you also... the lady and her baby have left now and you are sitting alone again... again notice how you are feeling and allow any emotions to surface...

When you are ready you see the shop open and you make your way inside... you find your way to the baby section... you see tiny little outfits, dummies, nappies... again allow yourself to feel anything that comes now without judgement... send love to yourself... there's no-one else around so let your emotions flow freely... this is a safe place for you to feel anything you are feeling... you might like to pick a jumpsuit up... feel the fabric in your hands... as you do so you feel a knowing within you that one day your baby will wear this jumpsuit... you can enjoy this moment if it feels safe to do so... feel the weight and the warmth of a baby in your hands now... notice how this feels... send love to yourself and to the baby and to the jumpsuit and all of the other items in the baby section of the store... it is safe to want these things... it is okay to feel any emotions you are now feeling... savour the feeling of holding that baby... spend a few moments now enjoying this feeling...

When you are ready, carry this feeling with you as you leave the store... knowing at any time when you are feeling sad you can re-visit this feeling to remind yourself of the possibilities... the deep knowing within you... breathe a deep breath down into your lungs, as you become aware again of the sounds outside of the room... gently bring them back into your focus, and then start to acknowledge the sounds in the room around you. Notice if it is warm or cool... become aware of where your body is meeting the chair or floor... of where your feet are resting on the floor. And breathe life back into your physical body... allow some gentle movement into your hands and feet. You might like to wiggle your hands and feet, your mouth. And when you are ready you can open your eyes.

*I can choose
to be the parent
I want to be.*

CHAPTER FIVE
BELIEFS ON YOUR ABILITY TO BE A PARENT

Write down all of the things that you are worried about with being a parent. Your list may include items from above, or anything else that comes up for you. If you can, explore ten positive reasons you have for being a parent as well. If you can think of more, I urge you to write more.

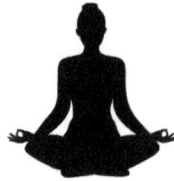

Meditation: for ability to parent

Our ability to be a good parent can be a big fear for many people, particularly if there haven't been good role models in your own life. My belief is we can choose to be the kind of parent we want to be. We can make a conscious decision to follow or not follow those that have come before us. We can take complete responsibility for who we are, and how we parent. This meditation focuses on being a good parent and is suitable for both men and women.

Find a comfortable position for this meditation. You might like to lie down with a pillow under your head and a nice warm blanket. Once you're comfortable, become aware of your breathing. Bring your breathing deeper... breathing deeply... right down past your lungs and into your abdomen. Then slowly and gently, let the breath back out. Notice how the breath fills your lungs completely... right down to your tummy, deep... deep breaths. And notice how gently it turns and slowly leaves, out through your mouth... continue to breathe in this way.

Become aware of a gentle feather, brushing the top of your head. Notice that where the feather touches, any stress or tension gets swept away. Feel the feather coming down over the top of your head, and around the back of your head... down over your forehead, your eyebrows, your eyes... your nose, your cheeks, your ears... across your mouth and around your jaw, down to your chin. Feel all the stress start to leave your body with the touch of that feather. Feel the feather go down over your neck... in between your shoulder blades, and down across your shoulders... down your arms, past your elbows down to your wrists and to the tips of your fingers. Feel the feather gently brush down past your chest, down your back and your sides, across your tummy... around your buttocks and into your legs. Feel all the tension just be swept away as the feather gently brushes down your legs, past your knees, your calves and into your ankles... down to the tips of your toes. Notice how heavy and relaxed your body feels.

Now see yourself standing in a beautiful park... smell the fresh green grass... feel the sun on your face, a gentle breeze... you hear the happy laughter of a child, and as you look around you recognise your child running towards you... notice how you feel seeing this beautiful being you created coming towards you... notice how you respond... do you lift your child into the air... perhaps you crouch down next to him or her, as they show you something exciting they found in the park... notice how you talk, the tone of your voice, the words you use... notice how easily you connect with your child, how natural it feels to hug and love them...

As you run around and play with your child, you notice they fall over onto the grass and they look to you to see what happens next... notice how you reassure them... provide comfort... show your child they are safe and loved... notice how effortlessly you care for this little being... how easy it is to love them...

You play for a little longer and your child picks up a stick off the ground and throws it at you... they think they are playing but you know it could hurt someone... notice how carefully you respond... how easily you find it to provide discipline in a caring and loving way... notice your child listen and take your words in, a lesson learnt in a way that is empowering and heart felt...

When you are finished playing for the day, you pick your child up and carry them towards home as they chat happily to you about the day and all of the exciting things they saw at the park... all of the fun they had with you... beautiful memories created between you and your child...

As you see yourself bath your child and tuck them into bed that night... notice how you feel... how capable you are of caring for this little human you helped create and bring into the world... spend a few moments enjoying this feeling...

When you are ready, become aware again now of your breathing. Take a few deep breaths, down into your tummy... and gently let them out. Become aware of where your body meets the floor, perhaps at your heels, or the backs of your legs... Your buttock and your back. The backs of your arms or your hands... And the back of your head. Just give your feet and your hands a gently wiggle, as you feel the life reawaken in you. Become aware of any sounds in the room around you... as you gently wake up. When you are ready you can open your eyes, ready to face the day and all the wonderful things it could bring.

I take responsibility
for my energy
and my emotions.

CHAPTER SIX
EMOTIONS AS ENERGY

There is a saying 'mind your own energy'. We are not taught a great deal about our body's energy system, and unless we go looking for this information, we may never know it.

Are there other areas of your life that you can identify where you see yourself as a victim or hard done by? You don't need to judge yourself here, simply become aware, take the steps to process these feelings, so you can change your vibration.

Identify the areas and write about these.

_____

_____

_____

_____

_____

_____

_____

_____

_____

_____

_____

_____

_____

_____

_____

Create a gratitude list. Make this a daily ritual.

_____

_____

56

_____

_____

_____

_____

_____

_____

_____

_____

_____

_____

_____

_____

Become aware every day of when you complain or judge. Simply acknowledge these thoughts and stop them in their tracks. Have an affirmation you can use at these times such as:

"I forgive myself for this thought, I'm choosing to let it go and view this person/situation from a place of love instead."

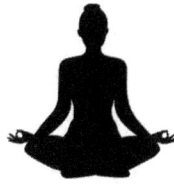

Meditation: for support

A lack of support can be a big fear for a lot of women during pregnancy and motherhood. This could be a result of being a single mum, perhaps your own mother is not around or not supportive. You may have a partner and yet still feel unsupported. It might be from not having friends that have children yet, or any other number of reasons. There is a saying it takes a village to raise a child, and this is true to a degree. Feeling unsupported for long periods of time can take its toll physically and emotionally. This meditation focuses on identifying the support you do have and creating a feeling of support by connecting to your own inner strength and divine source, or whatever it is you hold faith in.

Lie comfortably with your head rested on a pillow, use a blanket if you need too, to keep warm. Become aware of your breathing and observe how it starts to slow down as you begin to relax. Start to deepen your in-breaths, deep down into your abdomen, and just as slowly… release the breath as you exhale. Concentrate on your breathing for a few moments, slowly in… and slowly out… Feel any tension starting to leave your body. Starting at the tip of your head… relax your face and down your neck. Relax your chest and your back… slowly down your arms. Let the relaxation travel down your spine… your tummy, your back. Feel your hips relax… your buttocks. Relax down through the tops of your legs, over your knees, your lower legs and your feet… to the tip of your toes. Notice how relaxed your whole body feels, heavy against the floor or chair.

In your mind's eye, see yourself standing in a field. It's a beautiful field… you can smell the fresh flowers… feel the green grass soft under your feet… the sun is shining in the blue sky and you feel the warmth on your skin… there is a refreshing cool breeze that gently lifts your hair… you raise your face to the sky…. Eyes closed… Holding your arms out… notice how safe you feel here… how free… spend a few moments here simply enjoying the silence… your own company… feeling completely supported by all of the elements of nature… standing tall and strong… open to possibility… allow joy to fill you… peace… know there is nowhere else you need to be right now…

When you are ready you open your eyes… you sense someone standing near you… they are safe… supportive… as you turn to face them, simply notice who they are. This might be someone in your life now, someone who was previously in your life… or maybe they symbolise the person you would like in your life… they ask you now what you need. Take your time in replying… let any answer that comes to mind flow from your lips free of judgement… it's okay to want help… it's okay to want to feel supported… take your time and tell them everything you need in your life…

When you have finished, let your mind wander to the people who are in your life… those who do support you. It might be a partner… a parent… a friend… a colleague… they might support you in big ways or small… as you think of each person that supports you in some way, see them join you in the field… try not to force this… just allow the ideas and thoughts to come… if you are having trouble thinking of people, try to imagine the type of person you would like in your life and how they would support you… it might be the supermarket worker that offers to carry your bags to the car… it might be a supportive neighbour that brings your bins in… as you think of more and more people that could support you in life, bring them into the field with you… take as long as you need here…

When you are ready, look around the field and see all of the faces of all of the people ready to support you… see them smiling at you, and smile back… send gratitude and love to every single person that supports you in any way, no matter how big or small…

As you thank each of these people they leave the field until you are standing there alone once more, but feeling loved and supported… you might like to sit down now in the field, and as you close your eyes gently, you become aware of a different kind of being nearby… a supportive being that is a direct connection to universal source… it might be a loved one who has passed, your higher self, an angel, God… any divine source you feel a connection to… as they take a seat in front of you they look you deep in the eyes and ask you what you need… again take your time replying… how can this divine source assist you… perhaps they can send you signs to guide you throughout the day… perhaps they can send you helpful people… maybe it's just an angelic hug in the times that are hard… spend as much time as you need now talking to this angelic being, this divine source…

When you feel ready, you thank the being for coming here to support you today and know they will be with you always… know that in the future you can take a few quiet moments to connect with this Divine source whenever you are needing help or guidance…as you prepare to leave the field, take a moment to acknowledge any guidance or messages you have received here today..

Notice your breathing now… Become aware of the sounds in the room around you. Gently wriggle your fingers and toes… Take a nice deep breath in and as you exhale, open your eyes.

It is safe
to examine
my emotions.

CHAPTER SEVEN
EMOTIONAL AWARENESS

Is there a reason you don't want to get pregnant?

This sounds like a very silly question, but we often have underlying fears, beliefs, or emotions that stop us from getting pregnant. Let's look at some very basic concepts.

If I told you, hypothetically, that you would definitely get pregnant if you:
- Cut out all processed foods.
- Lost weight.
- Chart your mucous daily.
- Practice daily self-care measures such as meditation, yoga and tapping exercises.
- Walked around the block every single day.
- Stopped smoking/drinking/any other unhealthy lifestyle choice.
- Stopped blaming anyone else and took complete responsibility for everything in your life.

… would you do it?

If you said no to any of these things, then you need to ask yourself why not? If the thing you want most in the world is to have a baby, why would you not take every possible healthy step to achieve it? There are a lot of perceived downsides to having a baby as well.

Here is a list of just a few that I have come across, but I'm sure there are many more:
- I will get fat.
- I don't want stretch marks.
- I will lose my freedom.
- I won't be able to travel.
- I will need time off work, I can't afford that.
- It will hurt (labour).
- It could go wrong, and that would be too painful.
- My partner isn't kind, I don't want that for my child.

1. Did you say no to any of the questions? If so, write these down and explore the reasons you don't want to do them; you might be surprised by the answers.

_____

_____

_____

_____

_____

_____

_____

_____

2. If you said yes to all of them, are you doing them already? If not, write down why you are not doing them, or if you really believe this is an honest answer, start doing these things every single day. If you don't, you have a block here and you need to explore that.

_____

_____

_____

_____

_____

_____

_____

_____

_____

_____

_____

_____

_____

_____

_____

3. Did any of the downsides of having a baby resonate with you? Do you have others? Write about this and be very honest with yourself. No-one else needs to read this, but it is important you process these feelings and beliefs.

My happiness
is my responsibility.

CHAPTER EIGHT
FINDING HAPPINESS BEFORE THE BABY

Many people think they will be happy once they have a baby. I did. We assume we are only unhappy because we are infertile. That having a baby will fix everything, and we will be happy, and our lives will be perfect. While for some people, there may be some truth in this, however for the vast majority having a baby may not bring the happiness you thought it would. Once the baby arrives, it's hard work, you're tired, there could be financial constraints, there can be arguments over family roles, or if you're single you might resent never getting a break.

It's important to find happiness before the baby.

Identify ways you are obsessing about pregnancy or fertility and write these down.

_____

_____

_____

_____

_____

Identify areas or causes of stress in your life.

_____

_____

_____

_____

_____

If you track your cycles, notice where they indicate a stress response.

_____

_____

_____

_____

_____

Have you put any areas of your life on hold anticipating a pregnancy or a baby?

Once you have done this, I want you to try something that might be very difficult and will likely take practice and perseverance. I want you to set your intention of a pregnancy, don't limit it to dates and times, write this down, and then let it go, and simply trust it will happen.

Then, find a new focus for your life that creates passion and excitement for you. It most likely will be something creative: singing, dancing, knitting, classes on something new like cooking, or learning a language. You want an outlet for your stress that you enjoy and look forward to. That makes you smile when you think about doing it. You might want to book a holiday, or go for that job promotion, or enrol in a course.

If you can include your partner in this passion even better, it will help take both your minds off the fertility issue, unite you together in fun and strengthen your relationship. This might be kayaking down a river or taking dance classes together. It might be setting a 'date day' every week or month, where you go out to the movies and to dinner. Romance will flow more easily and allow sex to be fun again and not a chore that divides you.

This will raise your energetic vibrations and take the responsibility off pregnancy for being your only source of happiness and create new avenues for happiness and igniting passion in your life. Often times, pregnancy is a happy side-effect!

Write a list of things that make you happy.
How often do you do these things? Can you start doing them more?

I remind myself
to breathe…

CHAPTER NINE
RELEASING STRESS AND GUILT

Your body will let you know when it's stressed. Recognising and observing the signs is really important for your cycles and your overall health. Tracking your cycle is a great way to also monitor your stress. If you find ovulation is getting postponed, your cycles are becoming irregular or non-existent, check in with your stress levels.

Answer the following questions.

What causes stress in your life?

_____

_____

_____

_____

_____

How do you currently manage stress? Is it effective? Healthy or unhealthy?

_____

_____

_____

_____

_____

In what ways does your body show you that you're stressed?

_____

_____

_____

_____

_____

What are some new ways you can start to manage your stress more effectively?

_____

_____

_____

_____

_____

Write a plan to check in daily with your stress (recognition is vital), and any unhealthy 'tools' you are reliant on. Now consider new ways to manage your stress level. Commit to at least three things.

_____

_____

_____

_____

_____

_____

_____

_____

_____

_____

_____

_____

_____

_____

_____

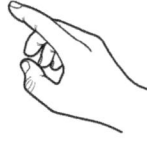

Tapping Script 3: for stress

This is a very quick tapping you can use if you are stressing out and feeling overwhelmed and need to calm yourself down quickly.

The karate chop point (KP): Even though I am feeling very stressed, I love and accept myself deeply and completely.

The karate point: Even though I feel overwhelmed at what I need to achieve today, I am okay.

The karate point: Even though I can feel my heart racing and it's difficult to breathe, I am supported, I have the tools in place to cope, I am okay.

Inner Eye (IE): I am stressed

Outer Eye (OE): am stressing out

Under Eye (UE): This is too much

Under Nose (UN): It's all too hard

Under Mouth (UM): I can't keep going

Collarbone (CB) *use fist*: I want to quit

Under Arm (UA) *use hand*: I can't do it all by myself

Top of the Head (TH): I'm feeling completely overwhelmed

Inner Eye (IE): I am okay

Outer Eye (OE): Breathe

Under Eye (UE): I am calming my body down

Under Nose (UN): My body is just trying to keep me safe and that's why my heart is racing. Include any other physical symptoms.

Under Mouth (UM): I am safe

Collarbone (CB): Breathe... *slow your breathing*

Under Arm (UA): I am okay

Top of the Head (TH): I'm breathing... *slower still*

*I am worthy
of a healthy
and loving
relationship.*

CHAPTER TEN
RELATIONSHIPS FOR FERTILITY

Are you currently in a relationship? If so, do you consider it a healthy relationship? Spend some time now doing some automatic writing about your relationship. Explore what is good, and what is perhaps not so good. Use these questions to help you write out your feelings.

Do you share the same ideas and beliefs around raising children?

_____

_____

_____

Do you agree on vaccinations, circumcision, discipline, schooling, religion?

_____

_____

_____

Do you want children equally?

_____

_____

_____

Do you harbour any doubts about your relationship or your ability to raise children successfully within it?

_____

_____

_____

If you are single, this is a good time to look at the type of relationship you do want, if you want one.

What will it look like?

_____

_____

_____

How will you treat each other?

_____

_____

_____

What aspects are important to you in a relationship?

_____

_____

_____

Will your new partner accept a child you have conceived via IVF?

_____

_____

_____

What role would a new partner play in the parenting of your child?

_____

_____

_____

*Being a mother
is my birthright.*

CHAPTER ELEVEN
SINGLE WOMEN AND SAME-SEX COUPLES

Being a single parent no longer has the stigma associated with it that it once did. Women can be proactive now and choose to start a family when they're ready. There's no more waiting around for Mr Right, or settling for Mr Right now. Single women or same-sex couples have an obvious fertility issue—a lack of sperm—which can be easily resolved using a sperm donor. Nevertheless, often these ladies don't have successful pregnancies straight away, and this causes them a lot of distress and loss of hope

Consider all of the questions, beliefs or judgements. Write about these, explore the beliefs and where they come from. Are they yours or some-one else's? Are they factual or a fear that may not eventuate?

I am grateful
for all of the options
available to me.

CHAPTER TWELVE
IVF, DONORS AND SURROGACY

1. If you are considering IVF, write about how you are feeling about this. Remember it is likely you will have very mixed feelings, so it's important to acknowledge the 'good and bad'. While you might feel grateful for the opportunity, you may feel anger and resentment at needing to do it, you may feel fear around the financial pressures, or any other number of emotions. Explore this in depth to process your emotions.

_____

_____

_____

_____

_____

_____

_____

_____

_____

_____

_____

_____

_____

_____

_____

_____

_____

_____

_____

2. If you are using a surrogate or donor, list your thoughts, beliefs and feelings around this. Consider the reasons for needing to use a surrogate or donor. What feelings does this bring up for you?

_____

_____

_____

_____

_____

_____

_____

_____

_____

_____

_____

_____

_____

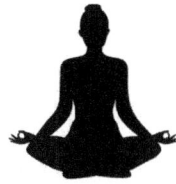

Meditation: for IVF

IVF is a process where eggs are removed directly from the ovaries and fertilised with sperm outside of the body to create embryos, and if they survive, transferred approximately a week later into the woman's uterus, or frozen if they are not being used straight away. Eggs can also be frozen without the use of sperm, which is becoming a common practice for women who are single and getting older but haven't yet met the person they want to have children with. This process is often used when there is a cancer diagnosis and treatment will likely cause the woman to become infertile. In this instance, often the woman will also need to find a surrogate to carry their future children, as pregnancy can be a significant risk factor for oestrogen dominant cancers returning. This meditation focuses on the first stage of IVF, where eggs are removed from the body, and is suitable for women going through IVF. This meditation uses a much shorter relaxation stage, so if you need longer to relax into the meditation, simply replace this section with a relaxation stage from another meditation.

Find yourself a comfortable place to sit or lie down, where you are warm, and your back is supported. Maybe sitting in a chair, or lying on the floor, with a pillow and a blanket. Once you are comfortable, close your eyes and take a nice deep breath in, filling up your lungs with fresh oxygen, all the way down to your tummy. And as you slowly release the breath, feel any tension leaving with it as your body relaxes into the chair or floor beneath you. Again, take another deep breath in, and as the breath turns to leave, feel it picking up your tensions and taking them from your body. Continue to breathe like this for a few moments, breathing in peace and relaxation and breathing out any tension or stress.

Now become aware of a beautiful rainbow light dancing around the top of your head. Swirling around. As it brushes past your skin it picks up any remaining tension dissolving it... and you feel it leave your body. Feel the beautiful vibrant colours of the rainbow, swirl around your head, down over your forehead... across your eyes, your nose, your ears, your cheeks, your mouth and down your jaw. Feel it swirl around your neck and around your shoulders, down both your arms, swirling round your wrists, and your hands and each of your fingers. Feel the rainbow swirling down your trunk... your back, your chest and your sides. Around your buttocks and each of your legs, slowly swirling down around past your knees, your calves, your ankles, your feet and each of your toes... As the tension leaves your body feel yourself relaxing heavily into the seat or floor, and the rainbow light just sits softly around you. Relaxing you, keeping you safe and warm, as you continue along this journey.

In your mind's eye bring your attention to your ovaries... see them full of healthy growing follicles... send calm and loving energy to both ovaries now... watch the follicles grow steadily... see an egg within each follicle.... Developing as it should... healthy and ready for life... take as much time as you need here.... Filling both ovaries with love... you might like to talk to your ovaries... thank them for the amazing job they are doing... for working extra hard this month... you might like to talk to the eggs that are growing... tell them how much they are wanted... how much you love them and are grateful to them for simply being... (You might want to do this stage several times during the start of your treatment before going to theatre for your egg collection. Skip to the re-grounding stage at the end until you are getting closer to going to theatre. When egg collection is near, move on to the next step of this meditation).

It is almost time to go to theatre and have your eggs collected... this is a good time to explain to your ovaries what is going to happen... tell your eggs they are being collected and they will be safe... not to be scared... that you will always be connected energetically throughout the whole process... if any of your eggs are too small ask them to begin maturing in preparation... if any are too large ask them to slow down and wait for pickup... explain to your eggs that fertilisation will take place soon and ask that they allow that to happen with ease... that they will be stronger once fertilised and a step closer to returning to your body... if you are having a fresh transfer let them know how many will be put back... if they are going to be frozen let them know that they need not be scared... that they are doing an amazing thing for you... and you will wait patiently to see them again in the future... send them a lot of love and gratitude now... spend as long as you need to here until you feel a deep connection with your eggs and your body feels loved and healthy... (again you might want to repeat this a few times leading to your egg pickup. Skip the next stage and go straight to the re-grounding stage. After your egg collection, move on to the next stage of this meditation).

Now that your eggs have been collected, in your mind's eye see them sitting in their petri dish, happy and full... growing as they should... see fertilisation happening with ease... let them know you are still here and waiting for them... remind them they are safe and very wanted... tell them they are loved... if you are having a fresh transfer let them know it's not long now and you will be re-united... if you are having embryos frozen tell them it's safe... that you will send them love the whole time they are frozen... that you will look forward to meeting them again in the future...that even though they are residing outside of your body for a short term, you will always be connected... always a part of you...

If your embryos are being frozen, you might like to do a meditation similar to this throughout the time they are frozen. If you are carrying your own embryos, you might want to move on to the next meditation now. If a surrogate is carrying your embryos for you, skip the next meditation and go to the meditation for surrogacy.

When you are ready, become aware again of the bright colours that have been resting around you, slowly coming back to life, surrounding your body, and bringing your awareness back to your physical body. Become aware of the chair or floor beneath you. You might like to wriggle your toes or your fingers, or your face. And just feel yourself again becoming one with your physical body. Take a nice deep breath in, and when you feel comfortable, that you are safely back in your body, you might like to open your eyes and just take a few moments before you get on with your day.

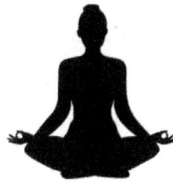

Meditation: for IVF embryo transfer

This meditation focuses on the next stage of IVF when you are having your embryos transferred into your uterus and is suitable for women carrying their own embryos.

Find yourself a comfortable place to sit or lie down, where you are warm, and your back is supported. Maybe sitting in a chair, or lying on the floor, with a pillow and a blanket. Once you are comfortable, close your eyes and take a nice deep breath in, filling up your lungs with fresh oxygen, all the way down to your tummy. And as you slowly release the breath, feel any tension leaving with it as your body relaxes into the chair or floor beneath you. Again, take another deep breath in, and as the breath turns to leave, feel it picking up your tensions and taking them from your body. Continue to breathe like this for a few moments, breathing in peace and relaxation and breathing out any tension or stress.

Now become aware of a beautiful rainbow light dancing around the top of your head. Swirling around. As it brushes past your skin it picks up any remaining tension dissolving it... and you feel it leave your body. Feel the beautiful vibrant colours of the rainbow, swirl around your head, down over your forehead... across your eyes, your nose, your ears, your cheeks, your mouth and down your jaw. Feel it swirl around your neck and around your shoulders, down both your arms, swirling round your wrists, and your hands and each of your fingers. Feel the rainbow swirling down your trunk... your back, your chest and your sides. Around your buttocks and each of your legs, slowly swirling down around past your knees, your calves, your ankles, your feet and each of your toes... As the tension leaves your body feel yourself relaxing heavily into the seat or floor, and the rainbow light just sits softly around you. Relaxing you, keeping you safe and warm, as you continue along this journey.

In your mind's eye bring your attention gently to your uterus now... see your uterus healthy, vibrant... see the endometrial lining thick and welcoming... see the colours vibrant and full of energy... talk softly to your uterus... let it know your embryos are returning soon and the important job it needs to play in accepting and carrying the embryos for you... spend as much time here as you need, gently preparing your uterus and lining...

Now move your focus to your embryos in their petri dish... tell them you are excited to meet them again shortly... that you are ready to welcome them home... that you have your uterus all ready to invite them in... to carry them and support them to grow into the baby you are so excited to meet... see your embryos healthy... calm... ready to be transported back to you...

Now bring your focus to your cervix... let it know that soon it will need to relax and open to allow a catheter to pass through with ease... so your embryos can be returned home... let it know it plays an important role in the process and you are grateful for its help...

You might like to do this meditation a few times in the lead up to your transfer. Skip through to the re-grounding phase until the time of transfer. During the transfer, you might like to do the following step.

It is time for your transfer... allow yourself to relax... the calmer you are, the more relaxed your embryos can be... the more welcoming your body will be to your embryos... as the transfer takes place, in your mind talk to your embryos... say hello... welcome home... I am so excited to see you again... we are ready for you...

Say anything here that feels right for you to establish a loving connection with your embryos. After your transfer, you might like to move on to the next step.

Your embryos are safely back home within your uterus now... see your embryo being welcomed into your endometrial lining... see it supported, happy... growing... healthy... see your lining vibrant with nourishment... talk to your body... tell it how loved it is for the amazing job it is doing... tell it how grateful you are... send love and health to your embryo and to your whole body... stay with this as long as you need to... come back to this meditation often throughout your luteal phase... encouraging your body and sending love every step of the way...

And when you are ready, become aware again of the bright colours that have been resting around you, slowly coming back to life, surrounding your body, and bringing your awareness back to your physical body. Become aware of the chair or floor beneath you. You might like to wriggle your toes or your fingers, or your face. And just feel yourself again becoming one with your physical body. Take a nice deep breath in, and when you feel comfortable, that you are safely back in your body, you might like to open your eyes and just take a few moments before you get on with your day.

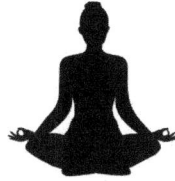

Meditation: for embryos being transferred into a surrogate

This meditation focuses on the next stage of IVF when you are having your embryos transferred into the uterus of your surrogate and is suitable for women not carrying their own embryos.

Find yourself a comfortable place to sit or lie down, where you are warm, and your back is supported. Maybe sitting in a chair, or lying on the floor, with a pillow and a blanket. Once you are comfortable, close your eyes and take a nice deep breath in, filling up your lungs with fresh oxygen, all the way down to your tummy. And as you slowly release the breath, feel any tension leaving with it as your body relaxes into the chair or floor beneath you. Again, take another deep breath in, and as the breath turns to leave, feel it picking up your tensions and taking them from your body. Continue to breathe like this for a few moments, breathing in peace and relaxation and breathing out any tension or stress.

Now become aware of a beautiful rainbow light dancing around the top of your head. Swirling around. As it brushes past your skin it picks up any remaining tension dissolving it... and you feel it leave your body. Feel the beautiful vibrant colours of the rainbow, swirl around your head, down over your forehead... across your eyes, your nose, your ears, your cheeks, your mouth and down your jaw. Feel it swirl around your neck and around your shoulders, down both your arms, swirling round your wrists, and your hands and each of your fingers. Feel the rainbow swirling down your trunk... your back, your chest and your sides. Around your buttocks and each of your legs, slowly swirling down around past your knees, your calves, your ankles, your feet and each of your toes... As the tension leaves your body feel yourself relaxing heavily into the seat or floor, and the rainbow light just sits softly around you. Relaxing you, keeping you safe and warm, as you continue along this journey.

In your mind's eye, gently bring your focus to your embryos in their petri dish... explain to them that it is time to be transferred into the uterus of your surrogate... tell them you are excited that a wonderful and generous person is happy to carry them for you... you might like to tell them how you are feeling about not being able to carry them yourself... but remind them they are very loved and very wanted... that you are always connected throughout this process... tell them your surrogate is ready to welcome them... that her uterus is all ready to invite them in... to carry them and support them to grow into the baby you are so excited to meet... see your embryos healthy... calm... ready to be transported to your surrogate... you might like to tell your embryo about your surrogate...

Bring your focus now to your surrogate... in your mind you might like to tell her what a gift she is giving you... send loving energy to her... see it fill her uterus with health and vibrancy... see this beautiful energy extend throughout her whole body... now see a connection from you to her... extend this energetic connection now to your embryos... see a triangular light connect the three of you throughout this process... spend as much time here as you need until you feel the connection... until you see all three of you calm and ready to proceed...

And when you are ready, become aware again of the bright colours that have been resting around you, slowly coming back to life, surrounding your body, and bringing your awareness back to your physical body. Become aware of the chair or floor beneath you. You might like to wriggle your toes or your fingers, or your face. And just feel yourself again becoming one with your physical body. Take a nice deep breath in, and when you feel comfortable, that you are safely back in your body, you might like to open your eyes and just take a few moments before you get on with your day.

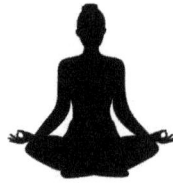

Meditation: for a surrogate

This meditation focuses on the next stage of IVF for a surrogate who is having someone else's embryos transferred into her uterus and is suitable for women acting as a surrogate for someone else.

Find yourself a comfortable place to sit or lie down, where you are warm, and your back is supported. Maybe sitting in a chair, or lying on the floor, with a pillow and a blanket. Once you are comfortable, close your eyes and take a nice deep breath in, filling up your lungs with fresh oxygen, all the way down to your tummy. And as you slowly release the breath, feel any tension leaving with it as your body relaxes into the chair or floor beneath you. Again, take another deep breath in, and as the breath turns to leave, feel it picking up your tensions and taking them from your body. Continue to breathe like this for a few moments, breathing in peace and relaxation and breathing out any tension or stress.

Now become aware of a beautiful rainbow light dancing around the top of your head. Swirling around. As it brushes past your skin it picks up any remaining tension dissolving it... and you feel it leave your body. Feel the beautiful vibrant colours of the rainbow, swirl around your head, down over your forehead... across your eyes, your nose, your ears, your cheeks, your mouth and down your jaw. Feel it swirl around your neck and around your shoulders, down both your arms, swirling round your wrists, and your hands and each of your fingers. Feel the rainbow swirling down your trunk... your back, your chest and your sides. Around your buttocks and each of your legs, slowly swirling down around past your knees, your calves, your ankles, your feet and each of your toes... As the tension leaves your body feel yourself relaxing heavily into the seat or floor, and the rainbow light just sits softly around you. Relaxing you, keeping you safe and warm, as you continue along this journey.

In your mind's eye bring your attention gently to your uterus now... see your uterus healthy, vibrant... see the endometrial lining thick and welcoming... see the colours vibrant and full of energy... talk softly to your uterus... let it know the important job it is about to do... the gift it is providing for another person... that this persons embryos are returning soon and the important job it needs to play in accepting and carrying the embryos for her... you might like to tell your uterus about the woman whose embryos you will be carrying... explain why she cannot do this herself... and how you are excited to work together to bring a new life into the world... spend as much time here as you need, gently preparing your uterus and lining...

Now move your focus to your embryos in their petri dish... tell them you are excited to meet them shortly... that you are ready to welcome them... that you have your uterus all ready to invite them in... to carry them and support them to grow into the baby that is so loved and wanted by its mother... see the embryos healthy... calm... ready to be transported to you...

Now bring your focus to your cervix... let it know that soon it will need to relax and open to allow a catheter to pass through with ease... so the embryos can be transferred into your uterus... let it know it plays an important role in the process and you are grateful for its help...

Bring your focus now to the woman you are being a surrogate for... in your mind you might like to tell her why you are happy to do this for her... send loving energy to her... now see a connection from you to her... extend this energetic connection now to her embryos... see a triangular light connect the three of you throughout this process... spend as much time here as you need until you feel the connection... until you see all three of you calm and ready to proceed...

You might like to do this meditation a few times in the lead up to the transfer. Skip through to the re-grounding phase until the time of transfer. During the transfer, you might like to do the following step.

It is time for the transfer... allow yourself to relax... the calmer you are, the more relaxed the embryos can be... the more welcoming your body will be to the embryos... as the transfer takes place, in your mind talk to the embryos... say hello... welcome to your temporary home... I am so excited to help bring you to your Mum... we are ready for you...

Say anything here that feels right for you to establish a loving connection with the embryos and to keep them connected to their mum. After your transfer, you might like to move on to the next step.

The embryos are safely home within your uterus now... see the embryo being welcomed into your endometrial lining... see it supported, happy... growing... healthy... see your lining vibrant with nourishment... talk to your body... tell it how loved it is for the amazing job it is doing... tell it how grateful you are... send love and health to your embryo and to your whole body... send this love beyond your body to the Mum whose embryos you are carrying... stay with this as long as you need to... come back to this meditation often throughout your luteal phase... encouraging your body and sending love every step of the way...

And when you are ready, become aware again of the bright colours that have been resting around you, slowly coming back to life, surrounding your body, and bringing your awareness back to your physical body. Become aware of the chair or floor beneath you. You might like to wriggle your toes or your fingers, or your face. And just feel yourself again becoming one with your physical body. Take a nice deep breath in, and when you feel comfortable, that you are safely back in your body, you might like to open your eyes and just take a few moments before you get on with your day.

*My past will
no longer determine
my future.*

CHAPTER THIRTEEN
ABUSE AND TRAUMA

Have you been a victim of abuse at any stage in your life? If it feels safe to do so, please write down this experience. Writing is an effective way of starting the emotional healing process. How did you feel during and after, your thoughts and reactions at the time, what you told yourself to cope? Writing this down will help you heal the negative feelings. If you haven't already, it is highly likely you will need professional help to work through your experience, and I would encourage you to seek this help.

*I can have a baby
while respecting
my culture and heritage.*

CHAPTER FOURTEEN
CULTURAL CONSIDERATIONS

What cultural considerations do you need to respect and adhere to?

_____

_____

_____

_____

_____

_____

Can you see any correlation with not becoming pregnant and the ideas outlined above?

_____

_____

_____

_____

_____

_____

_____

_____

_____

_____

_____

_____

_____

I am deserving
of more than
one child.

CHAPTER FIFTEEN
SECONDARY INFERTILITY

Explore the following questions and note any changes you can make to optimise your chances of a successful pregnancy. Consider how your life is different now to when you had your first baby.

You are obviously older, but what other factors are playing a role?

_____

_____

_____

_____

_____

What is your weight, diet and exercise regime like compared to last time?

_____

_____

_____

_____

Are you with the same partner, if so, has anything changed with him or his health?

_____

_____

_____

_____

_____

Are your cycles still the same, or are they changing?

_____

_____

_____

_____

_____

How are your stress levels, your sleep patterns?

_____

_____

_____

_____

_____

Other notes:

_____

_____

_____

_____

_____

_____

_____

_____

_____

_____

*I give myself permission
to grieve my loss
and to move on
when I'm ready.*

CHAPTER SIXTEEN
FERTILITY AFTER MISCARRIAGE, ABORTION OR A STILLBORN

- **Miscarriage.** A simple technique is to give yourself time when you won't be interrupted to sit quietly and bring your attention to your uterus. If you can, visualise your lost baby. This may be as a baby, as a colour, or simply as a feeling within your uterus. Out loud, or in your head, say all of the things you would have liked to have said to that baby. That you loved it, how much you wanted it, how much you still want it. Tell it it's okay to move on now and ask for its assistance and protection for any future babies.
- **Stillborn.** You can use the same technique as above, but this time visualise holding the baby in your arms to say your goodbyes, instead of in the uterus.
- **Abortion.** In the event of an abortion, whether you were okay with the decision or not, you can use the above technique to help yourself and your body let go of the emotions and move on. In this instance, you might like to tell your child your reasons for the abortion, knowing they are now a spiritual being and can understand this from that perspective, not that of a small child. You might like to explain why you made the decision, and that even though perhaps it is still affecting you now, you need to find peace with it, so you can move on.

Ask the baby you lost for assistance to bring another healthy baby into the world for you to love and cherish.

If you need further help with this, and if you need counselling to help you address these emotions, I would urge you to do so.

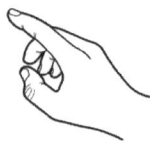

Tapping Script 4: for trying for a baby after having lost one

Often there are mixed feelings when trying for a baby after having lost one. Some people take relief from the fact they know they can get pregnant as sometimes that is a big step forward. Some people hold the fear that if they lost one already perhaps it will continue, or maybe there was something wrong with their baby that caused the loss and that could continue. Sometimes people feel guilt for wanting a new pregnancy when they have previously lost one. Your reactions and emotions could vary greatly during this time and may change from one minute to the next. That is the beauty of tapping, it is versatile, and you can use it as often as you need to as your emotions change. Some of the points below may not apply to you. It's unlikely you will feel all of these things at any one time, so please use the parts that apply to you and change or leave out the ones that don't. Your previous loss may have been due to miscarriage, stillborn, abortion or the loss of a child after he or she was born, which will also impact how you feel and how the tapping applies to you. For this purpose of this script I will simply refer to the loss as a loss, but you can make it specific to your circumstances if you find that helpful.

The karate point (KP): Even though I lost my baby, I love and accept myself deeply and completely.

KP: Even though I want another baby, I love and accept myself deeply and completely.

KP: Even though I want another baby after already losing one, I love and accept myself deeply and completely.

Inner Eye (IE): I lost my baby

Outer Eye (OE): that hurts

Under Eye (UE): I had hoped to hold my baby in my arms

Under Nose (UN): to watch her/him grow up

Under Mouth (UM): and that future has been taken away from me

Collarbone (CB) use fist: I lost my baby

Under Arm (UA) use hand: and that hurts

Top of the head (TH): but I still want all of those things

IE: I want to try again

OE: I want another chance

UE: but I lost one

UN: and I might lose another one

UM: and that's a painful thought

CB: it hurts to have lost one

UA: it hurts to know I may lose another

TH: I'm not sure how much hurt I can take

IE: was there something wrong with my baby?

OE: is that why I lost him/her?

UE: if so, what's to say it won't keep happening?

UN: I could keep losing them?

UM: there might be something wrong with all of them

CB: something wrong with me

UA: there's so much fear

TH: I don't know what's going to happen

IE: is it wrong to want another one?

OE: I can't replace the one I lost

UE: is it wrong to want to try?

UN: I feel guilty because I want to

UM: guilty and scared

CB: guilty and angry

UA: why did I have to go through this?

TH: wasn't infertility painful enough already?

Keep going as long as you need to, being as specific to your circumstances and feelings as you can be.

IE: it's okay to keep trying

OE: that baby wasn't ready to come into the world

UE: but I am allowed to keep trying

UN: perhaps there was something wrong

UM: but that doesn't mean the next one won't be healthy

CB: I am choosing to trust that it's safe to keep trying

UA: so, I let go of any guilt I'm holding on to

TH: I let go of the anger and the hurt

IE: I will look for the positives

OE: if I was pregnant once I can be pregnant again

UE: my body is learning what to do

UN: it is safe to hope I will bring a healthy baby in to the world

UM: I trust in the process

CB: I am allowed to want a baby

UA: even though I lost one

TH: it is safe to keep trying.

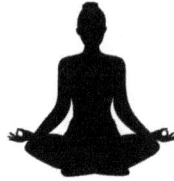

Meditation: for previous miscarriages

Experiencing a miscarriage is difficult. From the minute you know you are pregnant, you start to plan the life of that child. You might consider names, wonder if it will be a boy or a girl, imagine announcing their arrival to your friends and family, telling your partner you are pregnant. When a miscarriage happens, it can feel like the end of those dreams, and it's not always easy to let that go and move on to trying again. This meditation focuses on clearing the space where that baby once was and preparing the space for a new pregnancy. This meditation is suitable for any woman that has experienced a miscarriage.

Take notice of your breath. Take a deep breath in for 5, all the way down to your abdomen. Hold it for a moment… then slowly release the breath as you count to 5. Hold again and then breathe in again… counting to five… continue to breathe this way. As you breathe in, imagine a clear crystal rod from your crown chakra on the top of your head, extending down to your root chakra at the base of your spine. See the crystal rod changing colour with your breath as you relax, deeper and deeper. Violet…indigo…blue at the throat…green…yellow…passing your navel…orange…red…

Allow your mind to clear of all other thoughts. Let any fears… worries and tension dissolve from your body… gently floating out of the top of your head. Now see a glass box in your mind's eye. In this box is a bright flickering candle. Focus on the candle, as you allow yourself to be still. This is your time just to be. Silent… Still. Use the energy of the candle to re-charge your tired mind and body. Let the warm glow refresh you. Know that when life brings you fear or worry, you can focus on the candle and welcome stillness…

When you are ready let your focus shift from the candle to your tummy… going within… and as you look deep within your tummy you see the spirit of the baby that was once living there… the spirit is content, unaware he or she should have moved on… as you look lovingly at the beautiful little being that was yours, allow any feelings or emotions to come… there is no judgement here… no right way to feel… whatever you feel is perfectly okay and normal… spend as much time here as you need with this little being… you might like to tell him or her what your dreams for them had been… how much you loved them and wanted them… tell them you are sorry they couldn't stay with you…offer forgiveness for them leaving and ask for forgiveness for any fears you may have about what went wrong… forgive yourself for any judgements you hold towards yourself now… sending only love to yourself from this point forward… you might like to ask your little spirit baby if he or she has any messages for you… if it feels right to do so, you might like to ask this being if it will help you to conceive again, to bring you a new baby, and to watch over this baby as it grows and develops into a healthy baby… when you are ready, tell this beautiful little being it is time to move on… it's okay to return home… as you return your focus to the candle in your mind's eye, see it glow brighter and brighter and know your baby is passing through that light and returning home to where it belongs… and this place can be any place that feels right for you…

When you are ready, imagine the glow of the candle now moving towards your tummy… filling the space with a beautiful clearing and healing light… see the light move to any part of your uterus that needs healing… until all that is left is a fresh, clear space that is ready to welcome a pregnancy… spend as much time as you need here, preparing the space with love and healing energy…

When you are ready, bring your awareness back to your breathing… Take a deep breath in … 1,2,3,4,5. Hold it for a moment... Now release it slowly for 5... Again, holding at the end of the exhale. Now focus again on the crystal rod extending from your base chakra to your crown chakra. Starting at the base, imagine red light going to your feet, legs, hips and spine. See orange light coming up your abdomen... turning to yellow. Green light fills your heart... your lungs. Feel blue light going up to your throat... your neck and into your jaw. Indigo light awakens your ears... your eyes and nose. Now let a violet light bring sensation back to your whole body as it protectively wraps around you... and open your eyes when you are ready.

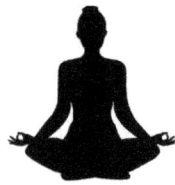

Meditation: for previous abortions

Making the decision to have an abortion is not always an easy one. Sometimes neither option feels right, but you have to make the best decision for you based on the circumstances at the time. I have worked with women that have had abortions who have experienced seemingly unrelated health issues later in life, which is the body's way of expressing the grief they may not have been able to express at the time. Sometimes there is an element of guilt, or anger. This meditation focuses on clearing the space where that baby once was and preparing the space for a new pregnancy. This meditation is suitable for any woman that has experienced an abortion, regardless if you felt it was the right option for you or not at the time.

Take notice of your breath. Take a deep breath in for 5, all the way down to your abdomen. Hold it for a moment… then slowly release the breath as you count to 5. Hold again and then breathe in again… counting to five… continue to breathe this way. As you breathe in, imagine a clear crystal rod from your crown chakra on the top of your head, extending down to your root chakra at the base of your spine. See the crystal rod changing colour with your breath as you relax, deeper and deeper. Violet…indigo…blue at the throat…green…yellow…passing your navel…orange…red…

Allow your mind to clear of all other thoughts. Let any fears… worries and tension dissolve from your body… gently floating out of the top of your head. Now see a glass box in your mind's eye. In this box is a bright flickering candle. Focus on the candle, as you allow yourself to be still. This is your time just to be. Silent… Still. Use the energy of the candle to re-charge your tired mind and body. Let the warm glow refresh you. Know that when life brings you fear or worry, you can focus on the candle and welcome stillness…

When you are ready let your focus shift from the candle to your tummy… going within… and as you look deep within your tummy you see the spirit of the baby that was once living there… the spirit is content, unaware he or she should have moved on… as you look lovingly at the beautiful little being that was yours, allow any feelings or emotions to come… there is no judgement here… no right way to feel… whatever you feel is perfectly okay and normal… spend as much time here as you need with this little being… you might like to tell him or her your reasons for having the abortion… how you felt about it then… how you feel about it now… tell them you are sorry they couldn't stay with you… ask for forgiveness for any fears you may have had then or now… forgive yourself for any judgements you hold towards yourself now… sending only love to yourself from this point forward… you might like to ask your little spirit baby if he or she has any messages for you… if it feels right to do so, you might like to ask this being if it will help you to conceive again, to bring you a new baby, and to watch over this baby as it grows and develops into a healthy baby, knowing there is no judgement from this Divine being… only love, forgiveness and understanding… when you are ready, tell this beautiful little being it is time to move on… it's okay to return home… as you return your focus to the candle in your mind's eye, see it glow brighter and brighter and know your baby is passing through that light and returning home to where it belongs… to a place that feels right for you…

When you are ready, imagine the glow of the candle now moving towards your tummy… filling the space with a beautiful clearing and healing light… see the light move to any part of your uterus that needs healing… until all that is left is a fresh, clear space that is ready to welcome a pregnancy… spend as much time as you need here, preparing the space with love and healing energy…

When you are ready, bring your awareness back to your breathing… Take a deep breath in… 1,2,3,4,5. Hold it for a moment… Now release it slowly for 5… Again, holding at the end of the exhale. Now focus again on the crystal rod extending from your base chakra to your crown chakra. Starting at the base, imagine red light going to your feet, legs, hips and spine. See orange light coming up your abdomen… turning to yellow. Green light fills your heart… your lungs. Feel blue light going up to your throat… your neck and into your jaw. Indigo light awakens your ears… your eyes and nose. Now let a violet light bring sensation back to your whole body as it protectively wraps around you… and open your eyes when you are ready.

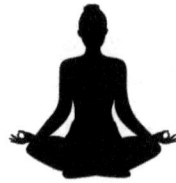

Meditation: for a previous stillborn

Having a stillborn baby is an incredibly difficult experience. Sometimes you know during the pregnancy that your child has passed, or it might be that you found out once they were born. It's important to give yourself time to grieve your loss, knowing the loss is a very real and significant one, regardless of how far into your pregnancy you were. It's not always easy to let that child go in these circumstances and move on to trying again. I've been told it feels like you are 'cheating' on the previous baby, or that you are trying to replace it. This meditation focuses on healing any judgements you hold around this and helps to prepare a space for a new pregnancy. This meditation is suitable for any woman that has experienced a stillborn.

Take notice of your breath. Take a deep breath in for 5, all the way down to your abdomen. Hold it for a moment... then slowly release the breath as you count to 5. Hold again and then breathe in again... counting to five... continue to breathe this way. As you breathe in, imagine a clear crystal rod from your crown chakra on the top of your head, extending down to your root chakra at the base of your spine. See the crystal rod changing colour with your breath as you relax, deeper and deeper. Violet...indigo...blue at the throat...green...yellow...passing your navel...orange...red...

Allow your mind to clear of all other thoughts. Let any fears... worries and tension dissolve from your body... gently floating out of the top of your head. Now see a glass box in your mind's eye. In this box is a bright flickering candle. Focus on the candle, as you allow yourself to be still. This is your time just to be. Silent... Still. Use the energy of the candle to re-charge your tired mind and body. Let the warm glow refresh you. Know that when life brings you fear or worry, you can focus on the candle and welcome stillness...

When you are ready let your focus shift from the candle to your arms that once held your baby for a brief time. As you look at your arms, you see yourself cradling the spirit of the baby that was once there... the spirit baby is content, unaware he or she should have moved on... as you look lovingly at the beautiful little being that was yours, allow any feelings or emotions to come... there is no judgement here... no right way to feel... whatever you feel is perfectly okay and normal... spend as much time here as you need with this little being... you might like to tell him or her what your dreams for them had been... how much you loved them and wanted them... tell them you are sorry they couldn't stay with you... offer forgiveness for them leaving and ask for forgiveness for any fears you may have about what went wrong... forgive yourself for any judgements you hold towards yourself now... sending only love to yourself from this point forward... you might like to ask your little spirit baby if he or she has any messages for you... if it feels right to do so, you might like to ask this being if it will help you to conceive again, to bring you a baby, and to watch over his or her sibling as it grows and develops into a healthy baby... when you are ready, tell this beautiful little being it is time to move on... it's okay to return home... as you return your focus to the candle in your mind's eye, see it glow brighter and brighter and know your baby is passing through that light and returning home to where it belongs... to a place that feels right for you...

When you are ready, imagine the glow of the candle now moving towards your tummy... filling the space with a beautiful clearing and healing light... see the light move to any part of your uterus that needs healing... until all that is left is a fresh, clear space that is ready to welcome a pregnancy... spend as much time as you need here, preparing the space with love and healing energy...

When you are ready, bring your awareness back to your breathing... Take a deep breath in... 1,2,3,4,5. Hold it for a moment... Now release it slowly for 5... Again, holding at the end of the exhale. Now focus again on the crystal rod extending from your base chakra to your crown chakra. Starting at the base, imagine red light going to your feet, legs, hips and spine. See orange light coming up your abdomen... turning to yellow. Green light fills your heart... your lungs. Feel blue light going up to your throat... your neck and into your jaw. Indigo light awakens your ears... your eyes and nose. Now let a violet light bring sensation back to your whole body as it protectively wraps around you... and open your eyes when you are ready.

*I am an equal partner
in our fertility journey.*

CHAPTER SEVENTEEN
WHAT ABOUT THE MEN

Traditionally, men are considered manly. They provide for the family, they are strong, and they can breed. So, finding out that sperm quality is not great for a man may not only be a big shock, but also a knock to their self-confidence and to the beliefs they held about themselves. Nevertheless, sperm problems can be a result of many different factors. Depending on the medical cause—if one is found—treatments will vary. You can help yourself by maintaining a healthy diet, regular exercise, quitting smoking, and avoiding drugs such as steroid use.

Do you have a physical issue affecting your fertility that you know of? Are there health and lifestyle change you need to make?

_____

_____

_____

_____

_____

_____

_____

_____

_____

_____

_____

_____

_____

_____

_____

_____

_____

_____

_____

*It is okay for me to
feel a range of emotions now
I'm pregnant.*

CHAPTER EIGHTEEN
WHAT IF I'M NO LONGER INFERTILE?

What about once you're pregnant?

So much focus is on the process of trying to become pregnant, that sometimes we can become defined by our infertility. So, once you are pregnant and no longer infertile, who are you? What about the support groups and all the friends you've made that are still infertile? How do those friendships survive if they are now feeling resentment towards you for achieving what they so desperately want? Conversations can become stilted, uncomfortable.

1. How would or do you feel when someone close to you becomes pregnant while you are going through infertility? Does this change your relationship with them in any way?

_____

_____

_____

_____

_____

_____

2. If you were to become pregnant, how would you want your friends to react and treat you? Is this different to what you wrote in question one?

_____

_____

_____

_____

_____

_____

_____

3. I want you to write two letters. The first is to the friend who has achieved a pregnancy while you are still trying. It can be a made-up friend if need be, you won't be sending the letter either way. Talk about how you feel and what you are finding difficult. Then talk about how you want to be, how you want your friendship to be, and how you are going to choose to feel and react in this scenario. The second letter is from you once you have achieved a pregnancy to a friend wo is still going through infertility. Repeat the process from the first letter but from this different perspective. Do these two letters give you some insight into both perspectives? Does it help to address some of the feelings that came up for you? Are there areas of your life you can apply what you have now learned?

Letter 1.

_____

_____

_____

_____

_____

_____

_____

_____

_____

_____

_____

_____

_____

_____

_____

_____

_____

Letter 2.

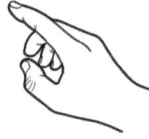

Tapping Script 5: for once you are pregnant

You might be wondering why there would be a need for tapping once you are pregnant. I mean that is the end goal, right? You must be over the moon, excited and elated. And you probably are all of those things. But often in addition to feeling very happy and grateful, there is an element of fear. After waiting so long and trying so hard, what if something goes wrong now? What if you lose the baby, or what if there's something wrong with it? What if you're not a good parent after all and there was a reason you weren't getting pregnant? What if your friends are jealous or resentful of you now you are pregnant and they're not your friends anymore. Who are you now you are not infertile? This could be a time of great joy and confusion. The tapping script is very general as you may be experiencing a few or many of the issues outlined. Use the ones you need to, skip over the ones you don't or change the words to suit your specific circumstances and feelings. Know it's okay to feel any emotions you are feeling. Nothing is right or wrong, it just is.

The karate point (KP): Even though I am so excited and grateful to be pregnant I am also quite terrified, but I love and accept myself deeply and completely.

KP: Even though I'm scared something will go wrong, I love and accept myself deeply and completely.

KP: Even though I'm worried my friends won't like me anymore, I love and accept myself deeply and completely.

Inner Eye (IE): I am so excited to be pregnant finally

Outer Eye (OE): but if I'm honest I'm also scared

Under Eye (UE): it took so long to get pregnant

Under Nose (UN): what if it doesn't stay?

Under Mouth (UM): what if there's something wrong with it?

Collarbone (CB) use fist: am I tempting fate trying to make this happen?

Under Arm (UA) use hand: maybe nature knew best

Top of the head (TH): what if it all goes wrong?

IE: I can't relax and enjoy it

OE: because I'm worried I'll jinx myself

UE: if I let my guard down something will go wrong

UN: it's all too good to be true

UM: what if I mess it up?

CB: what if I do something wrong?

UA: I couldn't cope to lose it now

TH: it would hurt too much

IE: what will my friends say?

OE: they are still infertile

UE: will they hate me?

UN: will they be jealous?

UM: should I tell them?

CB: is it rubbing it in their face if I tell them?

UA: is it wrong to not tell them when we've shared this journey together so far?

TH: I wish they were pregnant too

IE: what if all my friends disown me?

OE: I remember feeling jealous and angry when other people got pregnant and I couldn't

UE: what if they feel the same about me?

UN: what if they hate me now?

UM: this is really hard

CB: I just want to relax and enjoy it

UA: but I'm scared about so many things

TH: I don't want to jinx anything

IE: I feel confused about who I am now

OE: I have been infertile for so long

UE: my friends and support networks are infertile

UN: I'm in so many infertility groups

UM: should I leave those now?

CB: I can't tell them I'm pregnant

UA: this is really confusing

TH: I just want to be happy about being pregnant

IE: but I feel guilty for being pregnant

OE: and I feel scared that it won't all be okay

UE: what if something goes wrong and I am still infertile?

UN: it feels too soon to hope

UM: I want to be positive, but I'm scared to be

CB: what if something goes wrong?

UA: what if I'm not infertile anymore?

TH: what if I am?

Keep going as long as you need to, being as specific to your circumstances and feelings as you can be.

IE: there's nothing much I can do

OE: except hope

UE: I will be positive

UN: but realistic

UM: I know it's early days

CB: but I know stress doesn't help

UA: so, I'm going to keep myself calm

TH: I'm going to remember to breathe

IE: and I will be quietly hopeful

OE: realistic yet hopeful

UE: I will tell people when I'm ready

UN: and I will trust they will be happy for me

UM: as I'm sure I would be for them

CB: and if I am no longer infertile

UA: I can write a new story

TH: I can inspire others with my story

IE: because if I can get pregnant hopefully, they can too

OE: I have wanted this for so long

UE: and I want to enjoy it

UN: so, for now I will work through my worries

UM: I will be hopeful

CB: I will take care of myself

UA: and I will trust that everything will be okay

TH: I am so happy and grateful to be pregnant.

With acceptance
comes peace
and I am okay.

CHAPTER NINETEEN
ACCEPTING I WILL NEVER BE A MOTHER

You probably started reading this book with hopes of becoming pregnant. But if you've followed all the steps, done everything I've asked of you and yet you're still not pregnant, you may be feeling quite let down and defeated. If this is you, if pregnancy is no longer an option for you, I am so sorry. I had hoped for so much more than this for you.

So, you've accepted you will never be pregnant. What do you do now? First you grieve. Let yourself be sad, angry and anything else you are feeling. You get to feel however you feel and don't let anyone tell you what that should be or low long it should take. People will make suggestions like fostering and adopting, and these are valid options if they work for you. It is an involved process and, in some ways, can be as emotional and saddening as trying to become pregnant. It might be worth a conversation though. In no way do I believe if you choose to adopt or foster that you are any less of a mother, and I hope they could be options for you to explore in the next part of your story.

This isn't easy, so I send you a world full of love for this process.

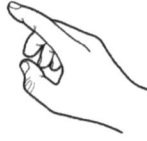

Tapping Script 5: for acceptance

At some point in this journey you may make the decision that you are done trying and accept that motherhood in the traditional sense is not part of your story. You might be okay with this decision if it has been a long time coming and you have had enough. It may be heartbreaking and a decision you never thought you would have to make. The tapping script below is a very general guide. Your feelings around this will be very unique to you. Some of what I write may feel completely aligned with you, and some may not even be in the ball park for you. So, use what you find helpful and change anything that needs to be changed. This script is more directed at people giving up on the idea of having a biological child that they carry.

The karate point (KP): Even though I don't want to give up, I know I have to, and I love and accept myself deeply and completely.

KP: Even though this is the hardest decision I will ever make in my life, I love and accept myself deeply and completely.

KP: Even though I know now I won't have a baby, I love and accept myself deeply and completely.

Inner Eye (IE): this hurts so much

Outer Eye (OE): how do I move on without a baby?

Under Eye (UE): I have spent so much of my life trying

Under Nose (UN): hoping

Under Mouth (UM): how can it be that I'm not a Mum at the end of it?

Collarbone (CB) use fist: that I never will be

Under Arm (UA) use hand: is this the right choice?

Top of the head (TH): should I try just once more?

IE: maybe the next time is the one

OE: but I can't live like that

UE: month after month not being pregnant

UN: it's too hard

UM: my life has been on hold

CB: I've given up so much already

UA: I need to stop now for my sanity

TH: for my health

IE: this wasn't the outcome I'd hoped for

OE: this wasn't the future I had pictured for myself

UE: I did everything I could

UN: and it wasn't enough

UM: and that hurts

CB: I tried so hard

UA: and I wished it was different

TH: but it's not and it's time to move on

Keep going as long as you need to here...

IE: I tried as hard as I could

OE: I know in my heart I gave it the best chance

UE: I couldn't have done any more

UN: it's time to put my energy into something else

UM: there are other areas of my life I have neglected that I would like to focus on now

CB: my relationship needs some TLC

UA: there's new creative projects I'd like to begin

TH: perhaps I could travel

IE: I might go for that promotion I had been putting off

OE: I know I will always have some sadness about not being a Mum

UE: but I'm okay

UN: it will all be okay

UM: I will take each day as it comes

CB: if I feel sad, I will let myself feel sad

UA: if I feel good, I will make the most of it

TH: and the good days will start to outweigh the difficult ones

IE: I am okay

OE: I can do this

UE: I can be okay with this

UN: I love myself and my life

UM: and I'm okay

CB: my life has other plans for me

UA: and it will be great

TH: I am great.

EMOTIONAL RESOURCES TOOLKIT

FORENSIC HEALING

I offer forensic healing sessions in-person or distantly. You can see full details at www.leahlloyd.com or visit www.forensichealing.com to find a practitioner near you.

EFT

Emotional Freedom Technique or tapping is a great tool for clearing negative beliefs and creating positive ones instead. You can visit www.thetappingsolution.com for more information, scripts and videos.

BOOKS

Using Positivity to Make a Better Life by Leah Lloyd.
The Secret Language of Your Body by Inna Segal.
The Low GI Guide to Living Well with PCOS by Dr. Jennie Brand-Miller, M.D.
All available from Amazon in e-book and paperback.

OTHER SERVICES

You may find the help of a naturopath, osteopath, chiropractor, acupuncturist or Chinese medicine beneficial. Ask around in your local area for practitioners that are recommended and others have found helpful in their fertility journey.

Despite doing the exercises throughout this workbook, perhaps you still have some lingering beliefs or feelings that you are having trouble shifting.

Here are some practical ways of clearing them once and for all!

Affirmations

Using what you have written is a great way to identify your emotions and beliefs that may need changing. Remember, if your new affirmation really doesn't feel believable to you, change the wording to 'I choose…' so that you can believe it, and it gives you an element of control back over how you are feeling. In time you will hopefully find you can remove the 'I choose' altogether.

Put your affirmations on pretty pieces of paper and stick them around the house where you will see them. I have mine on my bathroom mirror, but you might like to put them near your joggers if exercise is a focus for you now, or on the fridge door if you're trying to eat better, maybe on the back of the front door, reminding you to have a great day as you leave the house. Whatever works for you will be fine.

Here is the list of affirmations I have used for the purpose of this book, you might like to change these to suit your specific circumstances:

"I am not defined by my story."

"Today, I take back my power."

"I have the ability to heal myself."

"I connect with the healer within me."

"I commit to showing my body unconditional love and gratitude every day."

"I empower myself with knowledge."

"There are many healthy changes I can make to help me have a baby."

"It is safe to feel my emotions and to listen to what they are telling me."

"I acknowledge and respect my feelings as I work through them."

"I can choose to be the parent I want to be."

"I take responsibility for my energy and my emotions."

"It is safe to examine my emotions."

"My happiness is my responsibility."

"I remind myself to breathe…"

"I am worthy of a healthy and loving relationship."

"Being a mother is my birthright."

"I am grateful for all of the options available to me."

"My past will no longer determine my future."

"I can have a baby while respecting my culture and heritage."

"I am deserving of more than one child."

"I give myself permission to grieve my loss and to move on when I'm ready."

"I am an equal partner in our fertility journey."

"It is okay for me to feel a range of emotions now I'm pregnant."

"With acceptance comes peace and I am okay."

Essential Oils

I have used dōTERRA ClaryCalm to help manage cycles with good effect. A regular cycle is a good step in the right direction on any fertility journey. A few of my favourite oils (or blends) for fertility in women are:

Copaiba

Ylang Ylang

Jasmine

Melissa

Rose

Fennel

Yarrow

Geranium

*Emotional Support: Lavender, Roman Chamomile and Mandarin. (first trimester only)

Essential Oils for Sperm Health may include:

Frankincense

Basil

Cedarwood

Clary Sage
Geranium
Ginger
Juniper Berry

You can purchase dōTERRA oils through me at www.mydoterra.com/leahlloyd or if you are purchasing elsewhere, please ensure they are of high quality and pure, not synthetic, fragranced oils. I don't have any training in the use of essential oils, so please seek further advice before using them. There are plenty of resources available that can teach you how to use essential oils safely and effectively.

Bibliography

Anderson, KN. Ed. 1998, Mosby's Medical, Nursing & Allied Health Dictionary, 5th Edn. Mosby, USA.

The Fertility Society of Australia (2016). http://www.fertilitysociety.com.au/home/about/ [accessed 2/1/16]

Zegers-Hochschild, F., Adamson, GD., de Mouzon, J., Ishihara, O., Mansour, R., Nygren, K., Sullivan, E. and Vanderpoel, S. 2009. *International Committee for Monitoring Assisted Reproductive Technology (ICMART) and the World Health Organisation (WHO) revised glossary of ART terminology, 2009.* http://www.who.int/reproductivehealth/publications/infertility/art_terminology2.pdf?ua=1 [accessed 2/1/16]

www.ingramcontent.com/pod-product-compliance
Lightning Source LLC
Chambersburg PA
CBHW080952050426
42334CB00057B/2608